Peter McDonald

A DOCTOR'S AIM

MEMOIR OF A LONDON SURGEON

Copyright © 2021 Peter McDonald

ISBN: 978-1-8384269-2-7
Imprint: Hooked Books

All rights reserved. No part of this publication may be reproduced, distributed, or transmitted in any form or by any means, including photocopying, recording, or other electronic or mechanical methods, without the prior written permission of the publisher, except in the case of brief quotations embodied in critical reviews and certain other noncommercial uses permitted by copyright law. For permission requests, write to the publisher at hello@hookedbooks.co.uk.

These are the memories of the author, from his perspective, and he has tried to represent events as faithfully as possible. The author and the publisher do not assume any liability for loss or damage caused by errors or omissions.

Foreword	1
Preface	3
Chapter 1: The Drug Dealer	4
Chapter 2: The Ugliest Hospital In Europe	10
Chapter 3: The Smile On His Face	25
Chapter 4: A Lump In The Neck	39
Chapter 5: Early Years As A Doctor	51
Chapter 6: A Consultant Job Brings Tricky Patients	64
Chapter 7: How Management Makes Matters Worse	73
Chapter 8: Georgina And Her Lover	83
Chapter 9: A Twenty-First Birthday Party	93
Chapter 10: The Melting Pot	104
Chapter 11: Scribbling	116
Chapter 12: How My Patient Was Front Page News	131
Chapter 13: A Brace Of Victims	142
Chapter 14: How Overseas Visits Allow Me To Take Stock	155
Chapter 15: St. Mark's Hospital Comes To Harrow	168
Chapter 16: Why Medical Politicians Sing Out Of Tune	181
Chapter 17: Little People And Small Incisions	195
Chapter 18: A Journey To The USA	208
Chapter 19: From Medical Student To Surgeon	220
Chapter 20: Medicine, Music And Laughter	233
Chapter 21: Did He Save Lives?	245
Chapter 22: Covid-19	258
Chapter 23: Retirement And Beyond	272
Epilogue	280
Acknowledgements	282

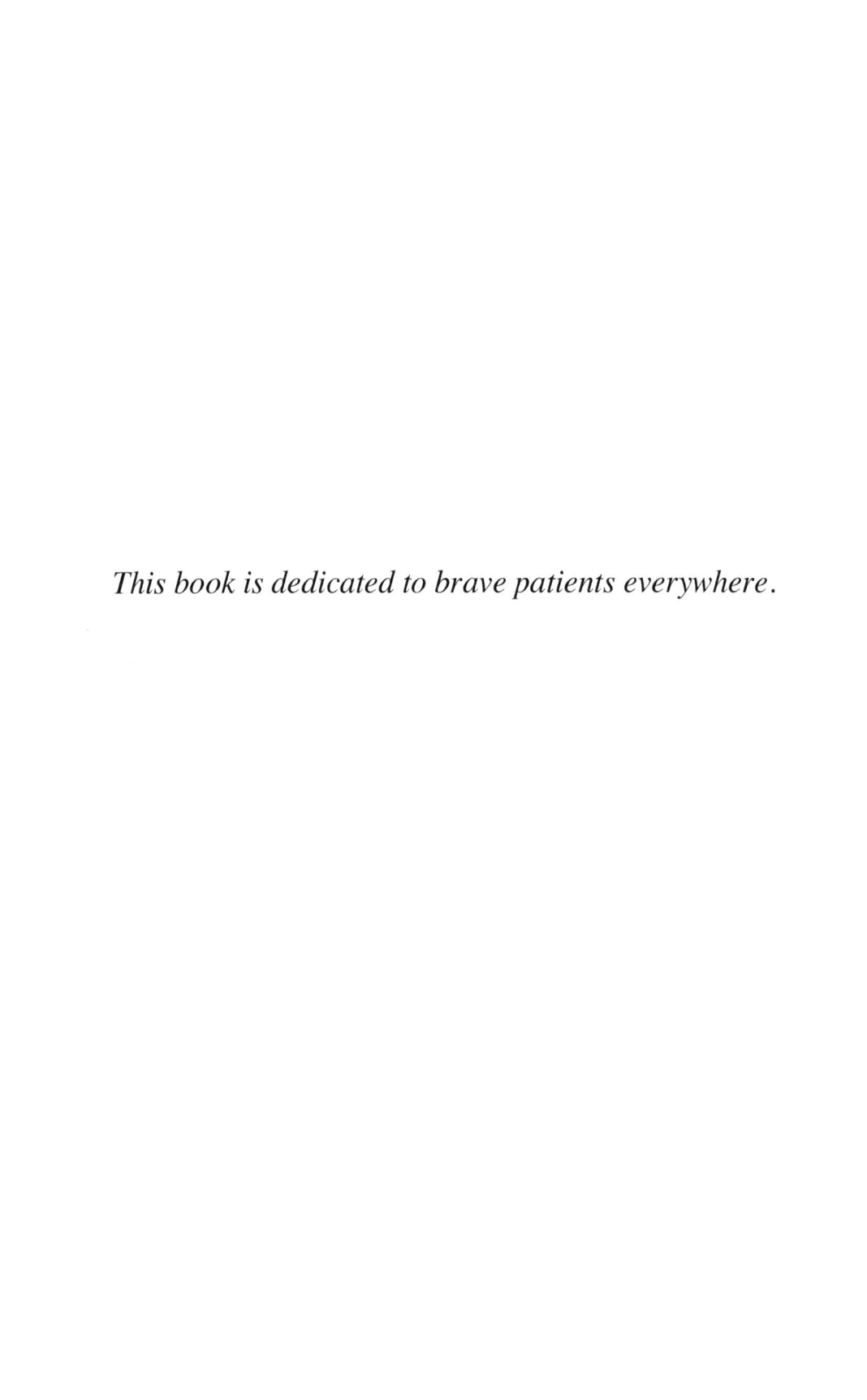

This book is dedicated to brave patients everywhere.

Foreword

I first met Peter McDonald fifteen years ago when I was referred to him by my GP. I had foolishly delayed getting a professional opinion, resulting in a belated diagnosis of bowel cancer. When Peter relayed this frightening and distressing news, he did so in concise and understandable terms whilst still displaying both sensitivity and a recognition of the mental trauma being suffered by my wife and myself. He outlined the optimum treatment plan and, in a short time, he had us feeling confident that this was a battle that could be won. A bond of trust and respect was created, which endures to this day.

In retrospect, I realised that he was at pains to understand me as a person and I am sure that all of his patients benefit from this holistic approach, as we all need to have our minds treated at the same time as our bodies.

I have, since that first encounter, had to consult my medical guru many times and he has saved my life on at least two occasions. He has also treated my wife and children, thankfully for less serious issues and I thought that I knew and understood him quite well. However, after having had the pleasure of reading *A Doctor's Aim*, I realise that I had only been scratching at the surface.

This book is a history of a remarkable and caring man. It gives a rare insight into the mind and experiences of a busy surgeon climbing the ladder from the bottom rung to the top. It also highlights many of the inner workings of our hospitals, both positive and negative, which hitherto have been a mystery to the mass of patients they treat.

This fascinating read illustrates the many and varied facets of the daily tasks of a compassionate surgeon. The predominant aim to care for patients, balanced with the desire to mentor and educate junior colleagues, for the benefit of all; the responsibility of leading a team with clear and pre-agreed policies and practices; the aspiration to communicate with the wider medical community to expand personal knowledge and skills coupled with the urge to share experiences with the worldwide community to question and secure medical advances.

The anecdotes expounded give the reader a picture of both the man and the attributes needed to survive and excel in the medical profession. They display the need for an ability to cope with the extraordinary pressures of making life and death decisions frequently. The humour and positive approach this necessitates is readily apparent. Peter's predisposition to see the amusing side is contrasted by the darker moments where the mental and emotional pressure of holding patients' and their families' lives in his hands is overwhelming.

We are all patients at some time in our lives and will have firm views, both good and bad, of the medical treatment and experiences we have encountered. However, only rarely do we have an opportunity to be invited in to see the 'warts and all' workings of the medical profession from the other end of the endoscope. In reading this very personal journey a reader will significantly enhance their understanding and appreciation of what it takes and, indeed what it costs, to provide such an invaluable service to humanity.

Andrew Kirshen
A patient
February 2021

Preface

A Doctor's Aim is a book about my life as a surgeon inside and outside of hospital.

It is about curing patients and sometimes failing to do so.

It is a book about why I chose this life and how my patients bravely face their hardships.

It is a book that charts the laughter and the sadness that goes hand in hand with that care.

It is a book about a hospital and the people that work in it.

It is a book about the follies of the administrative system that controls that hospital and the anomalies that stem from that control.

It is a book about desperate illness and the redemption of cure.

It is a book about how lucky we patients are today when we look back at how our forefathers suffered their surgical ordeals.

It is a book about the past, the present and the future of medicine and surgery with all their imperfections.

It is a book that might make you laugh and cry and think and dream.

But if Hippocrates could read this book, I hope it would make him just a little proud.

Peter McDonald
Hertfordshire, UK
April 2021

Chapter 1:
The Drug Dealer

❖

It was 10.30pm.
A Saturday night.
May 1992.

The body of the twenty-one-year-old was almost thrown off the trolley as it was pushed at high speed down the corridor to the theatre complex.

Surrounded by six nurses and doctors, the young man's face was hardly visible.

An Ambu bag supplying 100% oxygen from the cylinder under the bed was being pumped vigorously by one doctor as another squeezed hard the O negative blood bag being infused into the antecubital vein in his right arm.

'We're coming in now!' yelled the consultant anaesthetist as they crashed through the doors into Theatre 1.

'Patient number H365271... Unidentified male... aged 21!

Stab wounds to chest and right upper abdomen.

No visible external bleeding but gross abdominal distention and a pneumothorax, gas in the pleural cavity caused by the knife slicing into the lung, on the right side.

Systolic BP 70. No diastolic measurable.

Two litres normal saline given in ten minutes and now on his second O negative stat!

Saturations down to 84%!'

'Straight onto the operating table!' I shouted.

The patient's heart was not functioning properly and his tummy was very blown up, suggesting severe bleeding inside. As a result of this bleeding, the pressure of the blood was low so we began to transfuse further amounts of blood.

'We'll open him up immediately!'

Being warned of a patient with stab wound, I had scrubbed up five minutes beforehand with my registrar alongside me. As I lathered the iodine antiseptic soap into my hands and forearms, I reflected on the ordeal to come. Was I up to the task of holding this young man's life in my hands? I knew his very existence was on a knife-edge.

Perhaps there might be another surgeon who could do the job better than me, but I knew that at that precise moment I was the only person within ten miles who could save him.

The responsibility was almost crushing.

I would have liked to run away but I had trained long and hard for moments such as these.

Every fibre of my being told me to stay and face the music and do what I could.

I slipped my gown and gloves on and headed to the operating table. I felt someone rapidly tying up my gown behind me as I walked under the lights. The team was working well together.

The scrub nurse was ready with his instruments.

We prepped the chest and abdomen. We knew about the right-sided tension pneumothorax that was pushing the heart so far over to the left of the chest that no blood could be returned to it.

'Get that chest drain in quick!'

My registrar made a small incision between the fourth and fifth ribs on the right side in the mid-clavicular line and inserted a large number 20 French intercostal drain.

The sound of the air escaping from the pleural cavity was like some ghostly release of wind.

'Saturations markedly improving!' said the anaesthetist, encouragingly.

As my registrar began to tie in the drain with two silk sutures, I made a midline incision into the man's abdominal skin.

Through the linea alba, the white fascia between the rectus abdominis muscles, I cut straight into the peritoneal cavity.

Dark blood and huge clots belched out from the incision. It covered the towels and began to drip down onto my surgical boots.

'Suckers now! This is a massive bleed! Don't skimp on the O negative, please!'

'Second sucker now!'

My registrar strained over the table squinting at the blood-filled abdomen. So much blood. So dark. Almost impossible to see anything.

'Suck harder doctor!' I urged my assistant.

Together with two suckers we aspirated the blood into two huge plastic containers and scooped out handfuls of clots into the massive plastic bowl offered.

We were now in hot pursuit of the main bleeding point. There is usually, but not always, one culprit.

Once the bleeding vessel is found and sorted, control is normally achieved.

'Lights on the liver, please! Now!'

As I peered in with my registrar retracting the costal margin and applying the suction vigorously, I could see the problem immediately.

Three deep gashes into the right lobe of the liver were leaking blood.

One was particularly gushing.

Almost a fountain of blood.

'Packs now please!'

As I began to stuff the large abdominal packs onto the holes in the liver to create pressure and prepare to place some deep liver sutures, I heard frantic movements at the top end of the operating table.

Suddenly a fist punched onto the outside of the green towels covering the sternum which I had slung up to keep my field sterile. Then the unmistakable rhythmic violent shaking familiar to any doctor.

'CPR beginning at 10.47pm!' shouted the anaesthetist.

'No output! Asystole noted! Adrenaline given intravenously!'

'Peter, put some adrenaline directly into the heart if you can! If that does not work please open the chest and start squeezing directly!'

I finished packing the wound in the liver and passed a long needle through the diaphragm from below into the now lifeless left ventricle above.

I began to massage the heart directly from below the diaphragm.

'More chest compression! Thirty to two now! At 120 beats per minute if you can!'

The operating theatre was filled with the noise of men and machines doing just one thing.

Trying to save the life of the young man lying unconscious on the operating table.

Nothing else mattered.

The tension was hardly tolerable.

The deep concern palpable.

The theatre was now silent apart from the noise of the machines.

Nobody in the operating theatre cared as to how the young man had come to be there. He could be a sinner or a saint. It mattered not at all.

Another young man was rapidly losing his life.

We later learnt it was in the pursuit of drug wealth.

Somewhere his assailant was probably high on heroin slumped against a wall in a park.

For twenty-six minutes we battled to bring patient H365271 back to life.

Nothing worked.

More blood! More saline!

More adrenaline!

DC shock!

Nothing!

We had failed. And it felt very bad.

It was time to call it a day. Or rather a night.

'Withdrawing treatment at 11.23pm' I said quietly.

'Please certify death when you can Sally' I ordered my registrar.

'Thank you all for your hard work. Thank you. Shame it turned out this way.'

The grey body was now lifeless in a pool of blood, drips, tubes, and towels. My registrar and the scrub nurse were beginning to tidy up while I wrote up my notes. Both were in a state of shock.

Another lost future.

Could I have done something more to stop the bleeding? Should I have occluded the hepatic artery, the portal vein or some other major structure? I was feeling wretched. I wondered how the rest of the team were faring. As I finished writing up the report of the operation and the timeline of the cardiac arrest, I noticed some of the team were crying.

Perhaps some had sons of the same age?

Seeing sudden violent death so close up is more than even hardened doctors and nurses can cope with.

I turned away hoping they could not see my own tears.

I muttered something again about what a fantastic team they had been and wandered towards the theatre door.

**

Time for that most awful of tasks.

To break the news to the young man's mother and sister waiting in the relatives' room outside.

I plodded zombie-like along the corridor and held a mother's hand.

The sorrow and the tears were almost too much for me to bear. I began to weep a little too. I had done my duty but I had failed them.

I left them to a sympathetic nurse. The worst night of their lives had just started. It was a prelude to the lifetime of grief that they would feel until the day they too would die.

Later I drove through the traffic home to Hertfordshire not noticing that I was running many of the red lights.

Finally, I was in bed. But I slept badly, re-living every moment of the battle to save that young man's life.

If only I had done this or that manoeuvre?

What surgical trick had I missed?

It was a long dark night.

But not as long and dark as the endless night which that young man had just begun as he lay on his metal bed in the hospital morgue.

Chapter 2:
The Ugliest Hospital In Europe

❖

The hospital was larger than I had imagined.

I stood gaping at it for a long while.

Northwick Park Hospital in Harrow was more than a sight for sore eyes.

It was enormous, sprawling and in no way at all a pleasing spectacle.

Grey, ugly, and depressing, it gave out a tangible air of foreboding. I could not recall ever before having seen a building so unlovely.

I left my car in a parking bay, put a pound in the meter, and walked around to the main tower block. That morning it had been raining and the concrete walls of the hospital were stained with huge, black watermarks. It had created irregular patterns like one of those sinister psychological Rorschach Tests where you are expected to imagine a rampant gorilla or a bird of paradise.

Perhaps the builders of such a monstrosity had not been able to afford drain pipes when they had constructed it in the late 1960s? As the rainwater cascaded down its walls, I got the clear impression of a building that had been crying. Was it in sorrow? Was it reflecting the pain of the souls inside? This mystery added to the sadness of the scene.

This was Great Britain's National Health Service, where every cock-up of every project is never done by halves. I later learnt that a layer of marble cladding, which was to have covered the outside of the hospital to make it more attractive, had been omitted to save money as the project was over budget. Rumour had it that the architect had committed suicide when he saw the final result of his labours. Maybe that was just an urban legend but travelling as a man in search of employment, these first impressions added to my discomfort and apprehension.

I headed towards the central block in order to locate the senior surgeon's office. I had an appointment to see him but, despite being a mature man of nearly forty, I was really quite nervous. By any standard in the world, I was now a fully trained surgeon and it was time I had a permanent consultant post in the NHS. Although I considered I was long past my sell-by-date, getting a job was easier said than done. In my field of general surgery, specialising in the giblets, there were just too many surgeons like me chasing too few jobs. Some had thrown in the towel before now. Their faces not fitting. Their resolve failing. They had moved into other less competitive fields of medicine. Perhaps they were the sensible ones.

I had already applied for a couple of dozen posts and been interviewed for half of them without success. That day in England's bleak January weather I had no reason to think this visit to Harrow would yield a different result. My intention had always been to practice and live outside the capital so I had not applied for posts in London until this moment. But this job was particularly attractive and I was now getting desperate. In the back of my mind, I knew it was going to be hard to persuade my countryside-loving wife Christina to take our growing family any further into the metropolis than the M25.

Thoughts like this had finally led me to this horrid, box-like, grey building in Harrow. Although the hospital was little more than twenty years old, I entered it as if I was stepping into a mausoleum. Tentatively and with the humility that comes from frequent crushing defeats, I advanced towards that surgeon's office to begin my campaign.

I had no reason to know at that moment that the next thirty years of my life would be spent toiling in that grotesque edifice.

**

The office was on the seventh floor of the hospital. As I stepped out of the lift and stared through the dirty windows, I could see central London. Shafts of sunshine were trying to break through the cloud and I could just make out the Post Office Tower ten miles away. In the far distance the massive, monolithic features of One Canada Square, the highest tower block in Europe at the time, was just visible through the mist.

I found the office and knocked tentatively on the door. From behind it came an odd sound. It was of a man shuffling papers, a pause and then a grunt. Although I was just a minute behind the time agreed, it was another fifteen minutes before the door opened and a short man stepped out to greet me as if nothing was amiss.

Despite his reputation as a good surgeon, he was clearly rather shy. After a feeble handshake, we settled down to what turned out to be an extraordinarily awkward twenty minutes.

He started slowly.

'Thanks for coming up to see us before the short-listing date, Mr. McDonald. I hope you had a good journey despite the wet weather?'

'Er, yes. Thank you. I got here without much fuss,' I replied just before he launched in directly with his first real question.

'Good! And why do you want to come to work with us at Northwick Park Hospital?'

I took a deep breath in and wondered how to formulate an answer. Of course, I could not really say that I would be willing to work anywhere. Although I was exhausted by the process of being rejected, I had to make it seem that his hospital was special and that I had chosen it above all others.

In truth, I would have to lie.

'Well, er,' I began, 'because of its reputation, sir. Indeed, it is the only post in London that I have considered applying for as it appears to combine the business of a busy district hospital with the intricacies of medical research at the same time because of its renowned research centre. I might say it has a reputation second to none in this regard.'

Blah, blah, blah! I was beginning to regret sounding so fawning.

'Ah yes!' he replied sounding convinced by my sycophantic utterings.

Then there was a long pause. He was not much of an actor but he started nodding with an approving smile. He hesitated a few more seconds before continuing the interview.

'Now tell me about your surgical interests, Mr. McDonald if you would.'

Given the floor, I rambled on being as truthful as I could. After all, I could not say what I was really thinking. That this was just another interview in just another hospital in just another part of the United Kingdom. That I had already travelled up and down the length of the country in search of a job. During that irksome quest, I calculated that I had driven five thousand miles around Britain, spent hundreds of pounds in the process and applied for more than twenty posts. If anyone could write a guide to NHS hospital car parks and canteens it would be me.

It had all been so exhausting. All I now wanted was a place to put down roots, start my own practice, and build up a reputation for myself rather than for all the consultants who had trained me. As I sat in that small office on the seventh floor of that ghastly building, I looked out of the filthy windows at Harrow on the Hill. To save money the administrators of the hospital had not cleaned the windows. Through the grime I could make out the pleasing vision of Harrow School clinging to a grassy hill to the west. Founded in the sixteenth century, its fine buildings looked down at me and raised my spirits for a moment.

I learnt much later that it was said that the chairman of the committee that had set up this ugly new hospital was an old Etonian who was trying to get his own back on rival Harrow School. If that was true he had certainly succeeded, for the view looking down the hill to the hospital was grotesque, while the vista looking up at the school was very pleasant indeed. At least, I mused, I would get a decent view from my own office window if I was successful.

I was awakened from my daydreaming by another penetrating question.

'And what, if any, would be the benefits for Northwick Park Hospital if you came here, Mr. McDonald?'

'I would develop a first-class gastrointestinal surgery service with the help of the two gastroenterologists here already,' I retorted pompously.

'What about referrals outside your own declared special interest area? How would you handle those?'

This was a tricky question as it touched on vested interests. He was a vascular surgeon - veins and arteries - and what he was really asking me was to state that I would not interfere with his long, established referral practice. Even though I had been well trained in vascular surgery, I was very pleased to be giving it all up as it had never been quite to my taste. Too much blood all over the shop.

I gave as diplomatic an answer as I knew how.

He seemed content with my reply.

The questions dragged on a bit so I tried to make a light-hearted remark or two. My interrogator showed signs of wanting to laugh, but I guessed he was not much of joker himself. The most he could do was utter a chuckle or two. But oddly, I was warming to him bit by bit. He seemed simply a decent, dedicated and hard-working, straightforward sort of man and one who I was sure I could work alongside. I guessed he had few interests outside surgery. Later I discovered that this was indeed the case. He was in the hospital at 7am every day with the exception of Sundays and his patients and staff were utterly devoted to him.

'Is there anything I can tell you about the job that you may wish to know before we shortlist the candidates, Mr. McDonald?'

'Er, no, sir, I think you have answered all my queries,' I replied, relieved that the interview was finally at an end. As I left the room, he shook my hand more firmly than when I had arrived. I noticed a twinkle in his eye.

'I look forward to seeing you at the interview, Mr. McDonald.'

He paused for a moment as he wished the sentence to be fully appreciated by me. It was his first attempt at a joke that afternoon, for he let the words hang in the air for a good ten seconds before adding with a smile: 'Assuming you are lucky to get shortlisted, of course.'

I slunk down the stairs to the carpark and got into my old Vauxhall Carlton. As I drove out of the front entrance into the traffic I did not look back. It was probably just another wasted afternoon. Just like all the others I had made myself go through over the last few years. I was weary with it all so I did not allow myself a further thought about the awful-looking hospital whose walls wept under the eye of that handsome school on the hill.

***

When I got home to Southampton, my wife Christina asked me what I had done that day. I had spoken about going to Harrow to look at yet another job so I was able to answer her questions quite succinctly. It was not that I was particularly unhappy with my visit to London but I had simply lost the ability to get excited about the business of job hunting.

Anyway, we had more important things to think about as she was expecting her third child in four weeks' time. There was therefore no point in stimulating Christina's interest about a place she would probably never even have to visit.

As the days wore on, we were more and more concerned that this new baby was in the breech position. With my wife thirty-six weeks pregnant, and, after a failed attempt at turning the baby, it was surely going to come out the wrong way round. This increased the danger for both the mother and baby. That was the focus of discussion between husband and wife. Not the fact that I might be a candidate for a job at Northwick Park Hospital. In those days running up to the birth of Gabrielle any work details were very low down on the list of small talk.

Also, we had recently taken charge of what would be the first of many pets. Leo the kitten was half-Abyssinian and half-Siamese and it seemed that this mix-up of races had created a perfect feline storm as he was more than just a handful. Much of our time was spent helping Oliver, our six-year old, look after his new kitten while preventing Archie, aged seventeen months, from strangling it. On one occasion, we found the kitten had been posted into a drawer in a bedroom. We were sure Archie was the culprit but he appeared as surprised as we were when we found a very distressed Leo amongst the socks.

It was into this busy domestic setting that three weeks later a letter from Northwest London Regional Health Authority dropped onto the front door mat. It stated I had been shortlisted from the thirty candidates that had applied and I was invited to appear at interview. In the run-up to the delivery of Gabrielle I had all but forgotten about those forlorn tower blocks.

But now I would have to busy myself with Northwick Park Hospital all over again. Before the interview there would be many more people to see. It was thought important to press as much flesh as possible. I arranged yet another day's leave and drove up the motorway towards the capital.

I have always been very thorough doing the ground work before an interview. It was useful to know if there was a local candidate and if they were well thought of. It was also vital to have enough knowledge to avoid being wrong-footed in front of the interview panel. I was a seasoned campaigner and knew that if a committee of appointment was split between two favoured local candidates, it might be that an outsider would slip through and win the prize. This meant that, when this rare circumstance arose, I had to be in a strong position to be able to walk through that open door when the time came.

Despite it being an ordeal, I have always enjoyed going around the hospitals talking to those with the closest interest in a new appointment. The micro-politics of a hospital are as intriguing as any political party. There is much posturing on display to any outsider willing to listen. Frequently these informal meetings told me more about those I was trying to impress than they ever discovered about me. Often, I would be inappropriately taken into their confidence.

'Between you and me, Mr. McDonald...' a senior manager might whisper '...Mr. S___ does not yet know it but we are just about to cut his bed allocation as his budget is overspent.'

Then they would lean back in their chair with a look of great self-importance and suck the air in between their teeth and watch to see how impressed I was.

Another doctor, jealous of a colleague whose charms, skills, and hard work had allowed him to develop a thriving private practice alongside an NHS one, would offer an impertinent suggestion.

'Of course, Mr. B___ has always neglected his research and his NHS patients for the alternative. Do you know what I mean Mr. McDonald?'

They would stare straight at me for a few moments trying to detect my reaction. They would raise their eyebrows to the point of their receding hairline and cough pointedly. I felt it best to smile knowingly and say nothing much by way of reply.

In several interviews it was plainly obvious that many were trying to form premature alliances just in case I got the job. It was a long game and the process was intriguing.

After that second day of hustings at Northwick Park I raced back home to learn more of the impending epidural and our hopes of avoiding a forceps delivery. Secretly I was very pleased to forget about the hospital in Harrow and immerse myself in the worry over the baby. Actually, I was quietly confident that Christina, who had shed her first two bairns effortlessly, would have few difficulties even if the little darling was sitting the wrong way up.

***

Finally, the day of the interview came around. My best suit was dusted down and a shirt freshly ironed. As I headed north-east up the M3 I could not help but think that this would be just another wasted day.

I was bored with all this job hunting and I was almost ready to quit. Indeed, I had thought of abandoning my career in the rat race of medicine on three occasions. Once as a medical student while travelling in India I nearly threw in the towel to become a wandering hippie. Later, as a struggling surgeon, I had considered becoming a radiologist and, on another occasion, I had nearly joined a pharmaceutical company. Despite these rather feeble attempts at escape I had persisted. I may not necessarily possess the world's sharpest mind or even the slickest of surgeon's hands but I am a stubborn type who does not give up easily.

As I drove through the dawn rain, I thought about the ordeal ahead of me. Would it be just another unsuccessful day in a distant place talking uncomfortably about myself to a bunch of earnest strangers?

Probably.

I dreaded that awful feeling of yet another failure. I wondered that if it was repeated again today, would there still be enough fight left in me to pursue my ambition?

At the Regional Offices of the Health Authority all six interviewees had turned up. I knew them all well. We had spent hours together waiting our turn outside previous interview committee rooms and, during those hours we had swapped many stories, some intimate, some professional and some plain silly. Like me they were all dressed in suits except for the only girl present. Asha, a highly talented colorectal surgeon, had been a colleague of mine the year before at St. Mark's Hospital in City Road. Today she was on good form and, as she was bright and highly accomplished, I considered her the favourite for the job.

My turn for interview finally came at eleven-thirty. As I entered the committee room, I noticed something strange. There was a fifty pence coin on the carpet between me and the green baize table where the panel was seated. Should I stop to pick it up and offer it to the lay chairman to be handed in as lost property? Was this part of the interview? A form of initiative test?

After pausing for a second I decided to leave the coin where it was. I looked up at the panel and smiled sheepishly, recognising all present except for the chairman.

'Please be seated Mr. McDonald! Thanks for coming today. I am sorry to have kept you waiting so long. Let me introduce you to the panel, many of whom I know you have already met.'

The lay chairman was doing his best to make me feel comfortable but it was all a bit too gushing. Perhaps the panel were bored for it had already been a long morning. Indeed they looked exhausted. The chairman continued with his ramblings unaware that half of his committee was nodding off. He cleared his throat.

'I will ask Mike, Chief Executive of Northwick Park and previously of the Royal Navy, to open the batting.'

I had met the retired admiral in the days before. He was kind, charming and able and I had liked him immediately. In those days after the so-called NHS reforms in the early 1990s it was fashionable to appoint ex-military men to the NHS because of their organisational abilities. This practice was discontinued a few years later, as many seemed no more adept at coping with the impossible demands of the NHS than their predecessors. They could sink a battleship, perhaps, but not necessarily balance a hospital budget, where demand is perpetually out of control. There were a few exceptions to this rule and Mike was one of them. He charmed and he inspired.

'We see you have an impressive curriculum vitae, Mr. McDonald. A higher degree, a Diploma of the Royal College of Surgeons of England, time spent in America at the Cleveland Clinic and you have also been at St. Mark's too - the oldest bowel hospital in the world.'

'Er, yes, indeed.' I replied nervously, hardly recognising myself from the glowing description. But before I had time to gloat over my past achievements the ex-admiral continued ominously.

'We also note, however, that you appear to have been interviewed at many hospitals but have consistently failed to be appointed. I hope you do not mind me asking but why exactly do you think that is?'

The question took my breath away. I could see the panel begin to stir into life as they anticipated my reply. I paused for a moment before answering. How would I be able to pretend that these failures had not left scars? If I were on the committee the safest option would be to follow precedent and not touch a candidate like me with a barge pole. Although many of the candidates that morning were fellow veteran interviewees, I was certain there was not one who had been turned down as often as I had.

Part of the problem was that I had made my strong opinions well known in national medical newspapers. Although by then I had already notched up a respectable thirty-five scientific articles, I had also published by that time no less than four hundred personal view columns in the soft medical press. Many of these had been very critical of the medical establishment. I had used satire to point out its failings and the result had been that for every two amused and approving readers I had made at least one enemy. The problem for me was that these enemies were often in very high places.

I began my answer hesitantly in quite a different vein.

'My failure has been due to the fact that my own Health Region has no need at present of specialist colorectal surgeons and when I venture outside there is often a highly favoured local candidate.'

I was sensible not to add that these candidates were often nowhere near as well qualified as I was. The retired admiral looked up from perusing my CV.

'Don't you mean it is a case of the devil you know being better than the sarcastic medical journalist you don't?'

It wasn't going well. I tried to keep my composure.

'I suppose that might be one way of thinking about it but in my writings, I have always attempted to be constructive as well as critical.'

I wondered what the retired admiral was thinking of my rather weak defence. Fortunately, the chairman came back into the frame in conciliatory tone.

'Actually, someone yesterday showed me a copy of Mr. McDonald's latest piece in Hospital Doctor and, I must say, I found it well argued and really rather amusing.'

The ex-admiral was not to be pushed aside so easily. The tension was mounting in the room and I sensed that the whole committee was now wide awake.

'So, Mr. McDonald, even if you have achieved all that we read in your curriculum vitae, is there anything you can say today to us that might make us feel inclined to appoint you instead of the other candidates all who, I might add, have already achieved a great deal too?'

I sat miserably on the edge of my chair. The room seemed suddenly extremely hot and I was sure the panel were staring at the beads of perspiration that had appeared on my forehead. I could feel my sweaty palms clasped together on the table in front of me. I thought for a moment and realised that there was only one way to recover from the ambush the admiral had laid for me. I had to rebut the argument and then make a joke to diffuse the tension.

'Yes, sir. You are correct when you point out that I have been interviewed a great deal and have yet to secure a consultant post. But it certainly has not been for want of trying or from lack of practical and theoretical training.'

I hoped they could not sense the misery I was feeling admitting my failure. I had to keep going and with an added light-hearted touch. I continued by outlining in great detail that which I had achieved and what I could bring to the surgical team at Northwick Park Hospital in the decades to come. After labouring these points for some time, I took a risk.

'And indeed, I would do anything the committee asked of me to be appointed. I am so keen today that if it would help my cause I would be prepared to stand on this table, drop my trousers and sing three verses of Nellie Dean!'

The joke worked. The laughter was so loud that the candidates waiting outside wondered what had happened. I could see that even the senior surgeon was chuckling noisily.

The committee's questions thereafter were gentler in nature and the rest of the interview went well. Finally, I was dismissed and by the time I passed the fifty pence piece on the carpet on the way out, I was in high spirits.

The remainder of the morning dragged on as the last two candidates went through the same ordeal. After our individual torture was over, we would disappear to get a coffee before returning to hear to hear the verdict. In those days in the NHS, it was customary for all to be present at the announcement of the committee's decision. It was barbaric but perhaps it was character-building to eat humble pie five times out of six while watching a successful candidate leap for joy.

To be truthful, I cannot remember exactly how I passed those waiting hours that morning. Maybe I browsed in a nearby bookshop in Paddington or just walked staring into shopfronts? But I do remember climbing the stairs and rejoining my friends who were already milling around excitedly and taking bets as to whose turn it was that day. Was it to be my ex-colleague Asha or the accomplished chain-smoker from St. Mary's?

A few minutes later a door opened and a junior personnel assistant shouted out the finest phrase I had heard in my life to date.

'Would Mr. McDonald kindly step into the interview room to talk to the committee, please?'

Those words had been uttered to me only three times before in my medical life when successfully climbing each rung of the ladder. I would probably never hear them again because for most of us a consultant post in the NHS is a life sentence.

I could hardly believe it. It meant that my search for a permanent job was finally over. It had taken just under twenty-one years since I had begun as a medical student at University College London.

My marathon struggle had run its course and a belated victory was mine.

To this day, I recall every detail of what happened next.

As I entered the room the smiles of the panel members were broad and the congratulations generous and enthusiastic. Hands were shaken and pleasantries exchanged. It was all over in less than two minutes but as I left the room, I treated myself to the first of many indulgences that day.

As I passed the fifty pence piece, I bent down and swept it into my hand. I glanced back at the panel. One or two of them had noticed and were looking puzzled. Perhaps it had not been a test after all?

I smiled wryly back and gave them my best 'V for victory' before walking rapidly out of the room to begin my new life.

***

'Oh my God! We are not going to have to live in London, are we?' cried my wife down the phone.

Strangely, she had forgotten to congratulate me.

'No darling, not if you don't want to. We can easily live in a nice quiet spot within reach of Harrow and the hospital. Of course, I must be able to get to see the emergencies so it cannot be too far away. Maybe Pinner or Northwood?'

'But that's suburbia, darling!'

I thought for a moment and then conceded something to my wife that would affect me for the rest of my waking life.

'OK, Christina darling, we will live outside the M25. Somewhere rural and leafy, I promise you.'

But despite the inconvenience caused by living out of town I have never had any regrets that my heart suddenly softened.

The congratulations of friends and family were considerable that weekend. Many had despaired of me ever getting settled. A great weight had been lifted from my shoulders and I was looking forward to a new and exciting phase of my life.

As I made preparations to leave Southampton and move north to find a place for my family, my joy was redoubled when, a few days later, Christina gave birth to a baby girl by breech delivery in under two hours without the need of any artificial aid other than an epidural. Cuddling a new tiny baby is a feeling close to ecstasy, with the helpless creature's total dependence on you. A relationship so fundamental to the mystery and pain of living and dying.

For a few moments I was able to forget entirely about the difficulties of the preceding years and just dream of the challenges now to come. And with another baby to care for, what a joy it was going to be.

While I helped with the new infant, now called Gabrielle, by singing her to sleep the first night she got home, I was a bit sad that my ambition to succeed would, for a time, break up our comfortable home and later uproot them eighty miles to the north.

Yet as I looked into that baby's dark brown eyes, I saw my own reflection. Would she have ambition one day that would force her to make similar choices? I expected so. As I mused on the matter, I rocked her gently to sleep with the lullaby my mother had so often sung to me.

'Lula, Lula, Lula, Bye Bye!
Do you want the moon to play with?

The stars to run away with?
Lula, Lula, Lula, Bye Bye!'

I now knew that my own moon would soon be firmly looking down at that a ghastly concrete hospital in Northwest London where the rain made the walls cry, just like the baby in my arms as she struggled to sleep.

Chapter 3:
The Smile On His Face

❖

It was a clear June morning three months later when I looked out of the window of my small room in the hospital residence at the stirrings outside. I had been woken by my registrar with an early morning call. He was worried about a child who had come in as an emergency the day before under the care of the paediatricians.

'He's a lad of twelve with a four-day history of worsening abdominal pain and frankly, Mr. McDonald, I do not like the look of him. Could you come and see him with me before our operating list starts?'

I shaved and put on the suit I had packed at the weekend when I had left home. It was a bit crumpled but it would do the job. I needed to impress the locals during this first week at Northwick Park Hospital and, despite many years in preparation for this moment, I was apprehensive.

When I arrived on the children's ward, sister had finished the handover with her nurses. She peered quizzically at the new consultant.

'Mr. McDonald isn't it? Nice to meet you. We've heard a lot about you.'

She was almost certainly lying.

'Sorry to have to ask you to see this poorly little chap. He is a worry and his parents are frantic.'

'Not a problem sister,' I said, trying not to sound as nervous as I felt.

'Delighted to see if I can help. Let's go and examine him straight away, shall we?'

On this visit to the children's ward in my first week I knew I would need to be on my guard if I was not to fall short of my predecessor's high standards and clinical common sense. He had earned the reputation of being a solid, caring clinician and I would inevitably be compared with him. I was sure if I got this one wrong that my clinical ability, or lack thereof, would be broadcast around the whole hospital by lunchtime.

We moved into one of the ward bays and I caught my first sight of twelve-year old Steven. He was lying on a bed with an intravenous drip in his arm. His face was twisted with pain and his eyes were deeply sunken in their sockets. He looked very septic to me, with the classic features described by Hippocrates signifying an acute abdomen and peritonitis. That frightened, vacant stare was well documented by the Father of Medicine nearly 2,500 years ago on the small Greek island of Kos.

He was in bad shape.

He was dehydrated, listless, eyes vacant, and he was terrified to move.

'Hello, Steven, my name is Peter and I am the duty surgeon today. Sorry to hear you are not well.'

He looked at me suspiciously worried that I was yet another doctor who would hurt him.

I began my long list of questions. Do you have much pain at the moment? Where is it worst? How long has it been there? Does it radiate to any other part of your body? Does it hurt when you move?'

The poor boy took a long time to respond. Slowly he turned his large blue eyes towards me and with a despairing look whispered almost silently.

'It hurts me a lot! Down here!'

He pointed to the middle part of his stomach as I began to elicit his physical signs. He was pale. His pulse was fast and weak, his temperature was raised and his abdomen markedly distended. I gently pressed his abdomen but immediately he winced and I saw an expression of agony on his young, sweat-covered face. I knelt down on my knees and placed my stethoscope on his abdominal wall and waited for a minute or two. I heard absolutely nothing. The guts were silent, signifying a calamity within the peritoneal cavity.

I ran through the results of the investigations with the paediatric team. As I did so I glanced back at Steven.

He was truly frightened.

He needed reassurance and quickly.

'Never fear, Steven,' I said loudly to him. 'I promise I am going to get you better.'

I hoped he did not detect the worry I too was feeling.

But I now knew what I had to do and was quite certain we needed to act quite rapidly if we were to save this boy.

'Where are Steven's parents, sister?'

'They are in the office waiting for you, Mr. McDonald.'

'OK, let's get on with it. I think time is of the essence with this lad.'

The room at the end of the ward was occupied by a handsome woman of about thirty-five and a rather portly man staring out of the window. I could see the woman had been crying. I sensed that there was a lot of fear and anger in the air. When he saw me enter the man turned on me aggressively.

'You must be the surgeon we have been waiting for. What the hell's going on with my son? Nobody in this bloody hospital seems to have a clue what is wrong or how to make him better. He looks a lot worse than when he came in a couple of days ago. Last night one doctor even said he might have a bug which would respond to antibiotics, but they appear to be having little effect. What the hell are we supposed to believe?'

I waited a few seconds to let his anger subside before replying.

I then answered calmly but firmly. I began as gently as I could while maintaining control of the interview at the same time.

'Mr. Brown, Steven is very ill. That we know for certain. I think he has some catastrophe within his tummy which needs an emergency operation to establish what it is. Until we do that, I cannot be sure that all will be well.'

'But why can't you scan him to find out if he really needs an operation?' asked Mr. Brown.

'Actually, the ultrasound scan was inconclusive and further scans will just waste valuable time and probably achieve nothing further. The only decision we have to take now together in this room is to give me permission to proceed right away with an exploratory operation. My opinion is that he could die if we do not do this very soon.'

Steven's mother was in tears. Her husband continued sharply.

'But what if you're wrong, Mr. McDonald, and an operation is not helpful? Wouldn't that harm him further?'

These were the days before laparoscopy or quick CT scans. Nowadays it is possible after a preliminary scan to look in with a camera through a tiny incision and make a more accurate diagnosis. This is less traumatic to the patient.

But this was an earlier time and Steven's father was right. An unnecessary operation might tip the balance between life and death. Sometimes a surgeon has to have nerves of steel to advise seriously ill patients what to do. This time I knew I was on steady ground.

'Yes, Mr. Brown, it might be a risk but it is a risk we must take. Surgeons like me are always balancing up the probabilities of operations helping against their all too real dangers but in my view in Steven's case the choice is easy. I have a list starting in half an hour and I would like him to be the first on it if you give me your consent.'

Mr. Brown hesitated for a moment and turned to his weeping wife.

'What do you think Deidre?'

'Sign it Godfrey, for God's sake! Do what Mr. McDonald advises. It seems it is Steven's only chance.'

With that she began sobbing once more.

Godfrey took the pen and paper I held out for him and with an undisguised scowl scribbled an illegible signature on the paper. At the same time, he cursed under his breath.

He looked up at me and fixed me with a furious stare. The man was wracked with anguish and worry over the fate of his son.

'Look, Mr. McDonald, I don't care if you think you are the best consultant in the world, if Steven doesn't make it, I'll never forgive you or your bloody hospital!'

Without more ado he sat down and he too started to cry.

Many times, before and since I have observed how fear turns normally civilised men and women into irrational monsters. Polite, calm, mild mannered individuals can become aggressive and abusive even to those trying their hardest to help them. It is too often a case of shooting the messenger.

Sometimes I am reminded of Alexander the Great's reaction to the death of his close companion, and, maybe, lover, Hephaestion who died of alcoholic pancreatitis after one of their drinking sessions. Alexander's grief response was to crucify all Hephaestion's physicians as they had failed to cure his friend of his self-inflicted illness.

Luckily today we only get sued or struck off.

Understanding the genesis of this anger and controlling the response to it is one of the hardest and most skilful aspects of being a good doctor. We do not always get it right. But we must try.

When patients are ill and there are no beds to put them in or there is a lack of operating theatre time to carry out procedures, it is always the man or woman at the sharp end who bears the brunt of the ill-will. In today's society the tendency to blame the person trying to help seems to be a growing one and this can be expressed aggressively. Although most doctors find ways of rising above it, sometimes it can be very hard.

**

Steven was ready for theatre within twenty minutes, and soon after that was anaesthetised and prepared. As I looked at his swollen belly on the operating table, I pondered on what I might find inside. A perforated appendix, an incarcerated and strangulated hernia, a perforation from Crohn's disease or some congenital defect now manifesting itself after many years lying dormant? Any of these pathologies could be the cause of his sepsis.

I painted his abdomen with iodine from nipples to groin to allow me to expose, if necessary, the whole of the abdominal wall in preparation for the laparotomy. This odd word, first coined in the nineteenth century by a French surgeon, means 'cutting the soft parts'. I had no way of knowing if I would need a large, medium or small incision to cope with the disaster which I was sure was within.

On principle, initially I always make a small incision. As I say fatuously to my staff, much to their annoyance:

'I know how to make a small incision bigger but I have no idea how to make a big incision smaller.'

Of course, I expect them to be impressed by this wisdom but they never seem overwhelmed by it.

A wink from my anaesthetist told me that Steven's muscle paralysing anaesthetic was now working and also that he had adequate painkillers on board. A catheter had already been placed in his bladder to ensure that it would be collapsed when I entered the peritoneal cavity. It was there also to monitor the urine output accurately during and after the operation.

We were ready to start the laparotomy.

I made an eight centimetre incision in the midline vertically above, around and below the umbilicus. Carefully I cut down through the fascia. Beneath the peritoneal covering I could see some dark fluid bulging under pressure towards me. I incised into the cavity and, with a sucker at the ready, a torrent of black liquid began to be sucked through the plastic tube and into the reservoir. This liquid was a clear sign of a terrible mischief within.

Gently I began to inspect the small intestine. It was distended upstream but was collapsed close to where it enters the large intestine at the point where the appendix lies between the two. It was not just my hands and my eyes that told me what was amiss here. My nose had quickly picked up the scent of the putrefaction of dead tissue as we had entered the peritoneal cavity.

I took grim satisfaction that this smell alone meant that, without doubt, I had been right to order an immediate operation. Steven's life would now depend on what I could do and whether I had arrived inside his abdomen in time for his young body to mount an adequate inflammatory response after the surgery was complete.

I dissected a bit more and found the culprit.

A congenital fibrous band from the intestine to the back of the umbilicus had caused the calamity. Around this band a thirty centimetre long segment of small intestine had rotated and twisted, volvulus as it is called, and finally had become strangulated, losing its blood supply. It was lying on the right side of the abdominal cavity. Unmoving, black, paper thin with two or three perforations that were allowing small bowel contents to leak out bit-by-bit like oil from a stricken tanker.

I divided the fibrous band and delivered the intestine into the middle of the wound, trying hard to avoid further contamination. I checked the length of the remaining healthy small bowel at three hundred and fifty centimetres, meaning that Steven, at least, would have enough easily to live off afterwards. I isolated the forty centimetre segment of dead gut and packed off the rest with towels to protect the tissues from any more leakage.

I looked at my registrar and finally broke the tense silence.

'Worst is over, John. Let me assist you to do the resection.'

The next half hour was spent supervising my eager trainee perform something I had done myself three hundred times before. The mesentery with its blood vessels that supply the small bowel was divided between crushing clamps and the fresh, healthy and bleeding intestine's ends were sutured together with carefully placed dissolvable stitches. This is called an anastomosis, the joining together of two stomas, or mouths.

I watched the younger surgeon working, giving advice only when needed. He was doing a damn good job and I was quite sure he would soon be able to go solo. At the end of the procedure the foul-smelling black bowel was collected into a pathologist's pot for later analysis. The theatre started to smell sweet again while the abdominal cavity was washed out vigorously with saline and the wound closed in layers.

I relaxed for the first time since I had got up that morning. I called to my anaesthetist cheerfully.

'Is he stable?'

'Solid as a rock!' came the reply and from that moment I knew all would be well. In a previously fit youngster, the chance of any serious secondary complications occurring was now very small indeed. If only my own middle-aged immune system were as good as Steven's.

The tension of the last few hours was over. Everyone in the room was confident that the boy would survive and survive well. As we finished off the operation, the theatre was filled with light-hearted banter. In an operating room after a difficult procedure its occupants behave much as a rugby team in a communal bathtub after a hard game. Tales of previous brave surgical exploits are retold, and no doubt exaggerated, while stories recounted are liberally peppered with jokes.

Outsiders to this special world sometimes find this aspect of our behaviour odd, believing that surgeons and anaesthetists should be serious at all times. But humour inside hospitals is a rich vein made more relevant by the very nature of the life and death events that we see around us all the time.

I hope this feature of our work will never change. The day our politically correct masters legislate against humour may be the day we will all put down our scalpels. It is human nature to make light when a tense episode is over and it is right and proper to allow this to happen, however inappropriate it may seem to those who have never known what it is like to hold a human life in their hand.

As the banter continued that morning, it was an opportune time to discover a little more background about my new hospital. Surgery is a team game in which I was lucky enough, after all my years of travail, to be the captain. I could therefore turn the idle chatter to my own advantage and was soon learning of the foibles of colleagues from the more loquacious and less discrete members of the theatre team. Information gathering in this way one day might prove useful for me when problems in the hospital arose and allies might be needed.

After the operation Steven was in our surgical high care area for about twenty-four hours while the anaesthetists stabilised his fluid balance and his pain control. On the second day he was shipped back to the children's ward, where the ward sister and her girls clucked around him like mother hens who had just found a long-lost chick. That afternoon when I popped into the ward after my outpatient clinic, I noticed sister was wearing a smile that went from ear to ear. This was in stark contrast from her worried look of the previous morning. Now there was in its place an air of satisfied triumph tinged with what I judged was a measure of admiration.

'Mr. McDonald, I hope you don't mind me saying but I think you made a good call yesterday morning about Steven.'

'Well, thank you sister,' I said diffidently.

'We both looked at each other for a moment and then strangely we both blushed.

'Er, if your patients ever have need of me again…?' I mumbled as I walked awkwardly out of the ward.

***

I suppose I did not think much of Steven for the rest of that first week at Northwick. There were so many people to meet and so many things to sort out with my weekly programme that there was no time to spare a thought for anything else. My admirable secretary Lesley, whom I had inherited from my predecessor, needed to run through with me my working arrangements.

I discussed my open-door policy for colleagues, trainees, patients and relatives. She took in all my dictates without complaint. She was an impressive individual despite not yet being thirty. In the thirty years that have followed since that first meeting I have never ceased to thank my lucky stars that she is still my secretary. A tower of strength to me and my patients, she is loved by them all for her calm and reassuring manner. Indeed, she is given as many presents as I am by our grateful patients.

They often tell me how wonderful she is, even though most have only heard her voice on the telephone. Fortunately, jealousy is not one of my vices so I do not resent this fact but occasionally wonder how Lesley gets more credit for my operations than I do despite the fact she has never once been inside my operating theatre in nearly three decades working together.

In that first week there were clinics to run and several other very sick emergencies to sort out as well as a couple of colon cancers to operate on. As it was all rather busy, it was not until late on Friday evening that I finally got time to visit the children's ward again. My luck was in. It was sister's late shift so I was able to be brought up to date quickly and expertly.

'Progress good sister?' I enquired.

'Certainly, Mr. McDonald. He is a new boy and emerging out of his shell at an extraordinary rate. Come and see. By the way he has passed a bit of wind at last.'

Although this last bit of information must seem strange to impart to a colleague late on a Friday night, it was music to my ears. It heralded the end of Steven's post-operative ileus. This term describes the passage of time when the intestines sit passively, unable to function inside the peritoneum after an operation or a severe infection. The passing of flatus signified that all was now well and the guts and the anastomosis that had been fashioned by my registrar were functioning normally.

I have often joked with medical students that the best music I ever hear is not that which emanates from the car radio playing Elgar on Classic FM, let alone from my own second-rate violin-playing – it is the sound of a patient passing wind in the post-operative period.

'Good, very good, indeed, sister. Have you got time to pop in and see Steven with me? Are his family happier now?'

'For sure they are, Mr. McDonald,' she replied reassuringly.

So, in tandem we went to attend our sick boy.

In the third decade of the twenty-first century, it is rare to be able to do a ward round as a doctor simultaneously with a nurse in attendance, as nursing and medical practice on the wards have become disunited. This is not an improvement. The two groups now work independently and communication can be extraordinarily difficult. This separation of the disciplines is often at the expense of good team work.

However, that day nearly 30 years ago we, consultant and ward sister, were a true team as we walked into Steven's side ward.

Before I had a chance to examine the lad, two people jumped up from their chairs. Somewhat to my surprise I felt my arm being grasped very firmly by Godfrey Brown. Opposite me his wife was smiling warmly. Steven's father began first.

'Mr. McDonald, I want to thank you from the bottom of my heart for saving my son's life!'

'Thank you very much for your kind words Mr. Brown but, perhaps, it would be best if I looked at him first?'

His wife butted in as I moved towards the bed.

'Thanks for giving him back to us. You will see he is nearly his old self again.'

Indeed, they were right. Although Steven was lying a little stiffly, he looked a completely different boy from the one I had met just five days before. He was now able to grin at me for the first time and that evening I saw a sparkle in his eyes. I squeezed his hand gently.

'Feeling better Steven?'

'Yes thanks. A million times!'

'Still a little way to go but you will make it home by early next week if all goes to plan.'

'I did not really know I was so ill. I was sort of dreaming a lot but I remember you coming to see me before the operation. Now I feel myself again I cannot wait to get back to playing cricket.'

Steven and I then had the weirdest but most delightful conversation about his school cricket team. I listened to the details of the strategy that he, as captain, had adopted just a fortnight before his illness when playing his school's great rivals. Although he was still rather weary and a little puffed up, I noticed he displayed an extraordinary maturity for one of his age. This boy would go far.

'I think you had better rest a bit now Steven. See you on Sunday evening when I get back from my weekend with my wife and our own little people.'

I checked all his drugs and his fluid balance and thanked sister before waving at his still smiling parents. As I made my way home down the motorway that night, I was a man content. My first week as a consultant was over and already, I had been able to perform one of those little miracles that surgeons carry out from time to time.

It was a good start and I hoped a good portend for the future.

***

Steven left hospital four days later. He suffered no major complications. Later he told me he was fairly weak at first but was able to play cricket quietly fielding by the boundary just four weeks later. It was six weeks after he had resumed playing cricket that a postcard was delivered to me sporting a picture of a famous cricketing doctor with a huge beard. It was WG Grace.

On the other side Steven had written a message in a rather neat hand.

Dear Mr. McDonald,

Playing cricket again properly as Captain!
My tummy hurt at first but is now OK!
Thanks a lot!

Steven

Over the years I have kept many of these cards and letters of appreciation and one day I may write a paper about them for the British Medical Journal. It would be a contrast to the culture of complaining that seems to have so overtaken Western society in recent years. But few letters have given me as much pleasure as that postcard from that twelve-year old.

Occasionally I re-read these missives and they bring back many good memories of past patients. It is always said that a surgeon is only as good as his last operation. That may be true. Although we are intimately involved in the life and death dramas that make up the acute illnesses of our patients, we are rarely blessed with long-term relationships with them. We are like firemen putting out fires waiting for the next one to be lit. Unless the patients are unfortunate enough to suffer from recurrent disease, we do not often run across them again.

So it was that I never expected to hear from or see Steven unless he had a rare late complication of his intestinal operation.

It was therefore to my surprise and pleasure that I received a letter from him five years later containing a polite request. He wished to do a short period of work experience at Northwick Park Hospital with a view to taking up a career in medicine. I was delighted to help and a couple of months later he observed my team during a particularly busy week. Now a youth of seventeen with a keen brain, he marvelled at all he saw around him.

My house surgeon told me that he was on the wards at all hours to see the emergencies and to follow the clinical course of the patients. Indeed, he satisfied my main measure of intelligence in youngsters in that he never stopped asking questions.

A year later I learnt he had been offered a place at the University of Bristol's School of Medicine.

It was nearly seven years after that I received a neatly written letter from a Dr. Steven Brown.

Dear Mr. McDonald,

Although I have yet to decide which branch of medicine I will go into, I thought you would be interested to know that I am in my year of house jobs and am really enjoying surgery. Maybe I will try to become a surgeon? I am not sure yet.

I suppose all this started when you saved my life all those years ago. I cannot remember much about it now but my parents have often said how ill I was and how you did the trick!

Now as a doctor I seem often to be in a similar position as you were that day. I hope I can live up to your example.

This may be my last letter so I must say a final thank you to you and all who helped all that time ago.

Yours sincerely

Dr. Steven Brown MBBS

This letter is one of my greatest treasures buried deep in my archives. It speaks so much of what it is like to be a doctor and a surgeon in particular.

A patient on the edge of disaster plucked back from the brink by a desperate measure in miserable circumstances. Sometimes my patients ask me how it was that I had chosen unglamorous bowel surgery as a career. A life dealing with guts and smells, cancers and terrible infections. Why not something cleaner and more prestigious like cardiac, plastic or brain surgery?

There is no simple answer to that question.

I know all those other specialties have plenty of patients whose stories are not unlike Steven's. I know too that, although their work might be a little less agricultural than giblet surgery, there are plenty of sights and sounds equally as distressing and unglamorous in their fields as there are in mine. I also know that in those disciplines too there are many miracles to perform just like the one I was lucky to carry out on Steven that day in 1991.

After all is said and done, whichever branch of the healing art a doctor is committed to, it is the smile on the patient's face when they go home that is the real pleasure and goal of medicine.

Steven, I was told, had that smile when he climbed into his parents' car when they took him home after his operation that day in 1991.

**

From the memory of that smile alone I will never forget my first week as a consultant in that ugly hospital in north-west London.

But my pleasure at Steven's steady recovery from his operation would be quickly submerged as illness suddenly struck closer to home.

Chapter 4:
A Lump In The Neck

❖

A few weeks after I had begun my work at Northwick Park Hospital, I remember a weekend sitting and watching Christina breast feed baby Gabrielle. This little girl was an easy baby. She slept more or less to order and took her feeds regularly. She would grow into a beautiful, fair-minded woman.

I distinctly recall feeling extraordinarily happy as I gazed at my wife feeding her with the sunlight shining through the window opposite. It was an age-old scene of a mother and baby being at one. Christina was a fine-looking woman of some presence and as this was her third child, she knew exactly what she was doing.

She leaned back in the old nursing chair that was a relic from one of my great aunts.

I could see the perfect lines of her jaw and the lovely flow of her hair. The curve of her neck contrasting with the angle of her elbow as she supported the little one reminded me of the perfect lines of a Dutch masterpiece. It was a beautiful scene. Peaceful until she turned her head to listen for the toddler yelling upstairs. She leaned towards me and smiled implicitly suggesting I might want to investigate the noise above as she was fully occupied.

It was then I saw the lump in her neck.

I took a deep breath in and just stared at Christina.

Was it a true swelling I had seen in that brief moment or a shadow cast by the light coming around the curtain behind her?

Before I had a chance to register what I had seen I was given my orders.

'Go and see what he wants, darling,' she said quietly.

In a bit of a daze, I yomped upstairs and sorted out Archie. Aged twenty months he had managed to crawl out of his cot into the cat's basket and was keeping him company. I suppose he felt he was being ignored as the new baby was taking up so much of our time. But by playing with his feline friend, he had got soundly scratched. Hence the yelling and tears. I took him up in my arms and began a game to appease him before returning to the lounge. I sat down opposite Christina while Archie began to play with some toys on the floor.

'You've a lump in your thyroid gland, I think, darling. Probably just a physiological effect of the pregnancy but we may have to get it checked out sometime soon.'

She appeared alarmed for a moment and felt her neck.

'Not painful at least, Pedro.'

Ever since Christina and I had met, she had nick-named me Pedro. This was to differentiate me from her first husband Peter. Despite not having an ounce of Spanish blood in my veins, I am known by that name socially by most of our friends to this day and as Peter, or more formally, at work. This dual nomenclature has a geographical feature to it with the M25 delineating the change from Pedro to Peter. It means I always know from where any acquaintance comes.

But back to that pesky neck swelling.

'I might ask Simon to look at it on the ward next week,' she continued.

Christina was then a ward sister on our main surgical ward at the university hospital. She had been made a sister at twenty-three and was widely acknowledged to be a first-class manager of her staff and a very caring nurse. She was a meticulous woman who never stopped working and could spot any detail of patient care that needed changing. If the patient was right-handed why had the doctor not put the IV drip into the left arm? When the patient was being encouraged to drink plenty of fluids, it was useless for her nurse to put the water jug out of reach. If a patient was being urged to keep in touch with their relatives why was the phone placed on a table on the other side of the room?

When my time comes and I have a desperate illness I hope I have a nurse like Christina. Compassionate, thoughtful and tireless to improve the lot of her patients. A true guardian for those in distress. I had been impressed by her qualities when I had worked on the ward for the professor of surgery. She really stood out from the others both as a nurse and a person and she was much admired by both the medical, nursing staff and her patients.

But she had recently suffered her share of pain. When her first-born Oliver was still a baby her flighty husband Peter had left her for another woman. Perhaps he could not take the responsibility of a new baby or perhaps he felt sidelined? Although he tried to retrace his steps a few months later, Christina had been so hurt that she declined the offer. I flatter myself that perhaps her decision was influenced by the fact I had appeared on the scene by then.

I too had suffered personal miseries before we had first met. I had recently got divorced and was in a bad place. I had failed utterly in building a long-term relationship with my first wife who I had met at university years before. She was a struggling social anthropologist and I was a very junior doctor. Not a good combination perhaps.

Working frantically hard at our individual careers we had left no time for each other. In addition, I was subsidising her postgraduate studies and, although I was earning a reasonable salary, this was a source of deep frustration to me. There seemed to be no end to her need for funds for travel and research. Never a budget I could work to. I seemed always to be the giver and she the taker. An example of this one-sided arrangement comes to mind as I remember reading and correcting carefully her DPhil thesis but I cannot recall that she ever read mine.

We were both strong willed, fiery characters and we had drifted apart. Finally, the marriage had fizzled out. The decree absolute was a source of much regret and soul searching for me but I had to free myself from something I could no longer navigate.

Christina was attractive. Enough to make me want to do it all again, but would I succeed with another long-term relationship when I had made such a mess of the first one?

There was only one way to find out.

One day I had plucked up enough courage to ask her out to the opera in Southampton.

The Welsh National Opera was performing a couple of nights at the Mayflower Theatre in the town. It was Verdi's Il Trovatore. Giuseppe Verdi had read a play written by the Spanish writer Gutiérrez and had urged his librettist to create an opera of great drama. Together composer and librettist certainly succeeded. The union of Leonora's voice with that of Manrico in the Miserere scene is a sublime moment that always moves the audience. It was a grand night and a superb performance and we loved it. I remember looking at Christina transfixed in her seat and thinking that she was the girl for me.

This was the first in a sequence of events that would lead to me marrying her three years later. There were a few adventures to be had before that would come about. I think we were both very careful to make sure that the second time around would be different from the first.

Six months later she joined me for a couple of weeks when I was working in the USA. We toured the continent together. Jumping on and off planes and revelling at the incredible cityscapes and the geography of that huge country. We fell in love all over again. Much later, when we were in Australia visiting my twin brother Paul in Sydney, we were staying with a distant relative, a psychiatrist, who spoke his mind over dinner one evening.

'Why don't you marry her Peter? You obviously get on so well together. It seems damned obvious if you ask me.'

Trust a psychiatrist not to mince his words.

A chance conversation can change a life. Sliding doors and all that. This simple remark made me resolve that it was time to make a move but I waited until we had returned home and were in the routines of work again.

When finally, I asked Christina to marry me she was ever the rational ward sister. After all she had been left with a baby by her first husband without warning and she was determined that she would not make a similar mistake again.

'Can I have forty-eight hours to think about it Peter?'

I nearly choked on my pea soup in the hospital restaurant. Perhaps I should have chosen a more glamorous venue than the canteen to pop the question?

I was astounded by this two-day cooling off period but agreed to her request trying clearly not to show how much my masculine pride was hurt. But my patience was rewarded, presumably after detailed family discussions had taken place.

We got married without much fuss in the registry office in Southampton. Neither of us were churchgoers and, as we had both been married before, it seemed the most appropriate thing to do. A dozen members of the family were present including adorable Oliver, aged three. Then a honeymoon in London where we took in four shows and three museums over four days. It was April and it was cold but it was idyllic.

Not long after we married, we were back on Christina's ward working together again. I had rotated on to her ward for a further year of training in gastro-intestinal surgery. I remember a ward round with her when we were reviewing an old man recovering from an operation on his sigmoid colon. He was doing well and I thought he could be discharged shortly with Christina's help in organising various aspects of support for him.

'I think you might get home tomorrow, Mr. Williams,' I said confidently.

He smiled and looked pleased.

'Thank you, Doc,' he replied with a cheeky look in his eye.

His over familiar manner surprised me but I thought no more about it. Five minutes later I rushed off to theatre to start my operating list.

I later learnt that not long afterwards the old man had called Christina back to his bedside.

'Sister, I hope you don't mind me commenting, but I think that doctor, his name escapes me, you know the one who was with you on the ward round? I hope you don't mind me saying but I think he fancies you.'

Christina smiled sweetly and replied.

'That's very nice you should say that Mr. Williams. I think you may just be right. I hope so, anyway, as we got married a couple of weeks ago!'

***

Fast forward three years and it was on this same ward that Simon, a thyroid surgeon, had his patients. It was to him that Christina was referred concerning the lump in her neck. She saw him a week later.

He was very assiduous and examined her carefully. He was a cheerful optimistic surgeon who was much liked by everyone.

'He thinks it's just a simple benign nodule in my thyroid that ought to come out sometime before we have all made the move to Harrow,' she told me.

So it was that Christina had her operation two months later. Gabrielle was allowed to stay with her so that the breast-feeding ritual would not be too disrupted. She was back home the next day and I got some time off to help. Although her neck was a little sore, she was in good spirits and was coping well. Christina is a brave woman who always puts others before herself and never burdens those around her with more than is needed.

The clips came out the next Friday.

I had resumed my work at Northwick Park that week and on the Friday evening I got stuck in traffic on the motorway coming back from Harrow. I arrived back in Southampton about 8pm.

The children were all asleep except Oliver, now six, who needed to be read to.

We finally sat down for supper at ten but just as we did the telephone rang.

'Who can that be at this time of night?' Christina asked.

'Might be your mother finding out how you are?' I said.

Christina went into to the hallway to answer and I carried on with my meal. I could hear clearly.

'Hello, Simon, nice to hear from you.'

There was silence for a minute and then I heard a distinct sob. I found Christina slumped in a chair with the phone in her outstretched arm pointing for me to pick it up.'

'What's happened Simon?' I asked.

'Peter, I thought you ought to know straight away as the histology is back on the lump. I'm sorry to have to tell you over the phone but it has turned out to be malignant. Probably a papillary carcinoma or a mixed type and I am afraid Christina is going to need the rest of her thyroid gland out.'

The news hit me like a brick falling on my head. I have often had to break bad news to patients and have observed the devastating effect it can have on them. This was now happening to me.

No. This was now happening to us. Although I knew well that thyroid cancer was a much kinder cancer than the solid tumours of the gut that I would spend my life treating, cancer is still cancer. I also knew even when it arose in the thyroid gland it still occasionally had the power to kill eventually.

I grabbed Christina and held her close.

'Thanks Simon for telling us so promptly. It is a shock though. Can I ring you back in the morning?'

I replaced the receiver and held my wife to my chest.

I thought more of what I knew of this tumour. I knew that 90% of certain types of thyroid cancer could be cured. Others were much more lethal. But the price of success was a further operation followed often by radio-iodine treatment and maybe replacement therapy lifelong. But why Christina and why now? Was it the curse of the Chernobyl rain that had fallen on us five years before? Was it linked to the crisis of her sudden abandonment by her husband? Was it just bad lack or bad genes? Who can tell?

We cried quite a bit that night. I remember the image of a six year old watching us from the top of the staircase as we embraced each other in our fear and dread of the future. There was a quizzical, uncomprehending look on his face. I tried to explain it to him but it seemed better to simply hug each other and wait for the terror to pass.

The terror did pass as it always does but it was replaced by a feeling of constant unresolved worry always just under the surface. A worry able to break through at any moment of day or night. But we were busy people with responsibilities and life had to go on regardless.

And so it did.

Over the following few weeks, we planned our next steps. I would take compassionate leave from Northwick Park Hospital and Gabrielle would be weaned from breast feeding and put on the bottle. Christina would have to ready herself for a greater ordeal. When the day came for the total thyroidectomy, we were both prepared. Christina for the pain and me for the responsibility of looking after our little brood.

The operation went well but post-operatively Christina's calcium fell rapidly. I was fully aware that the parathyroid glands control calcium metabolism and that they are situated behind the lower part of the thyroid gland. Unfortunately, they are both tiny and very difficult to spot when operating but also their positions are not constant. I had often spent time trying to identify them when I had been involved in that sort of surgery. Not only can they be removed inadvertently but in the process of dissecting out the bulk of the thyroid gland their blood supply can be affected too. Then the glands fail and the calcium level in the blood drops.

'We have removed the rest of the thyroid,' said Simon to me the day after the procedure, 'and I am glad to say there was no residual tumour in it. I will get the pathologist to confirm that in due course.'

'That's very good news Simon,' I muttered.

'But the fact that the calcium is so low means that the parathyroid glands must have been taken along with the thyroid,' added Simon sheepishly.

'It is too early to say but that means that Christina will need both thyroid and calcium replacement medication for the rest of her life,' he continued.

So, the operation had achieved its purpose but we had a significant complication in having to keep the calcium in the normal range. We had understood the risks so were philosophical.

***

It was a blow to have suffered a permanent complication after an operation but no more than I had been forced to tell patients myself after surgery. All operations have both benefits and problems. Patients know that but always seek and expect perfection. Frequently they are disappointed.

I often joke that I have never done a perfect operation and that there is always room for improvement. Self-evidently a truism but somehow, we, surgeons, have failed to get this message across.

Take the example of an orthopaedic surgeon replacing a hip joint which has given the patient intractable, severe gnawing pain for many years. That surgeon knows that the same pain-relieving operation which will transform the patient's quality of life can result in substantial complications. It can result in asymmetry of leg length, infection of the prosthesis and even death from pulmonary embolism or concomitant heart attack. But as these risks are small the operation is deemed worth undertaking. Indeed, joint replacement must be one of the greatest boons to modern civilisation and demand for it in all its forms continues to grow.

The task that modern society has to address is how to reconcile these conflicting outcomes. We all want these pain-relieving miracles but we do not welcome the complications that may occur when we try to attain them. When complications do arise, the patient may look around for someone to blame.

One of the stresses of modern medicine that faces any practising doctor is this criticism. This may be in the form of a complaint or legal action leading to a civil or even a criminal court. Cynically I have often said that we live in a world today where those who do things leave themselves open to censure from those that do little. This is more true of surgeons than other doctors as their work clearly may both save or change lives in dramatic ways.

But surgeons can harm as well as cure. The stakes are high and our medical intervention is often imperfect. Patients' expectations may exceed often what is biologically possible. There seems also an in-built inability for society to recognise that health systems will never be comprehensive enough to guarantee perfect access for everyone at every moment in time. Prompt treatment sometimes is not possible.

The analogy with the airline industry, so beloved by commentators when they are highlighting safety in medicine, is all very well but it must be understood that, in many health services at unscheduled moments of emergency need, demand completely outstrips supply. It can be likened to several planes trying to land on the same runway at the same time. It does not work well. And it certainly is not safe. Mistakes and complications will follow.

The consequence in Western society is to attack the doctor by litigation to gain financial compensation. The problem today is that both the frequency and the cost of these attacks on the medical profession have grown exponentially. Yet there is no evidence to suggest that doctors are practising less safely than they did in former times. Indeed, quite the reverse is probably the case.

Because of the threat of litigation doctors in the UK must belong to a medical defence group that has the ability to pay out a sum in compensation to a damaged patient. This cover may be third party cover but mostly it is comprehensive, much as it would be for a car. This arrangement is called claims-made or occurrence-based cover.

At present in England the Common Law of the land means a claimant must prove that the doctor or the surgeon has been negligent. To receive compensation, they must show they have been wronged either through poor counselling or by a poorly conducted procedure. These torts, or wrongs, are debated in and out of the courts often years after the event. The result is that society has set itself up for expensive conflicts that often end with unsatisfactory outcomes. The medico-legal industry has grown huge in recent years and governments seem unable to control its rise. For the NHS the cost will soon reach £10 billion per annum.

When I was a young doctor, I paid £25 annually for my compulsory medical defence cover. Nowadays the government pays for all of my NHS liability but if I had to pay it myself my NHS cover would cost

£20,000 and for my private practice another £10,000. The system is close to being unsustainable.

In a publication recently it was calculated that one-third of the cost of NHS operations carried out in the high-risk specialty of neurosurgery was apportioned to cover these medico-legal risks. That proportion will continue to grow and eventually the cost of covering that risk will be so great that all operations in high-risk specialties will have to be curtailed. Obstetrics, plastic surgery, spinal surgery, obesity surgery and much of orthopaedic surgery will be the first disciplines to be put out of action.

If there is no widespread reform of the system many of the gains that medicine and surgery have made in the last one hundred years will be lost. A case of not only shooting ourselves in our feet but in our hip joints and many other important organs as well.

This was one of the reasons that I got myself on the board of one of the medical defence organisations (MDDUS) because I wanted to understand it all. But I also wanted to help where I could.

But I have digressed and I must finish the story of that lump in the neck.

**

Christina recovered from her ordeal with a brave smile. A smile with which she continues to charm everyone around her to this day. With or without a thyroid gland Christina makes everyone she meets feel happier. A rare character who moans never, criticises rarely and blames very few.

My ordeal after her second operation was to look after the children on my own for a while. It seemed I had been sentenced to hard labour, but I quickly learnt many of the tricks of childcare. I realised the importance of having everything to hand and to plan ahead. I coped with the chaos of the little people as best I could, often falling unconscious into my bed when I had finally got them all to sleep.

When I visited Christina in hospital, who was herself suffering and looked quite rough, I would say:

'Darling, you look great considering!'

She would smile weakly at me and replied:

'You look like death warmed up!'

Such was our exhausted marital rapport.

A short course of radio-iodine ablation treatment meant she had to be distanced from the children for a further fortnight. She got used to her new life of tablets and frequent screening blood tests and outpatient visits.

Her illness had been a lesson for me as both a doctor and a relative. When the hammer blow of a diagnosis falls, reason may be the first victim. The fear of the unknown may make a relatively small risk seem very great. As a doctor I know my job is as much to reassure my patients as it is to attempt to cure them. I have often told those with cancer that they are starting a long and difficult journey but that I will be with them all the way to guide them. I also tell them that they are not alone in that journey in that thousands have trodden the same path before them and I have looked after many who have survived the dangers encountered on the way.

Somehow this simple analogy of being on a journey reassures and calms them.

For Christina, like all cancer sufferers, the end of her journey with cancer involves sitting in the waiting room of life to see if the cancer returns. Many choose deliberately to put the problem to the back of their minds so they do not have to dwell on the memories of their diagnosis and their fears of recurrence. Others need to talk about it often to control these fears. There are many coping strategies and one-size does not fit all patients.

Nearly thirty years on, I write this on a sunny balcony on an Ionian island in western Greece. The view from the villa looking back to the mainland is one of the most beautiful seascapes I have ever seen. Christina is free from recurrence of her cancer. Her thyroxine level is normal and her serum calcium manageable. She is lean, fit and unstoppable.

The lump I saw in her neck that day thirty years ago, when she was feeding Gabrielle, cast a dark shadow for a long while but thankfully it did not prevent us enjoying many, many times when the sun has shone as it is shining here in Lefkada today.

Chapter 5:
Early Years As A Doctor

❖

With Christina's illness sorted and my consultant job in the bag, I was no longer a trainee. I was set fair for the rest of my working life.

I could plan.

I could invest in building my clinical service and my reputation.

If I wanted a thriving practice, I would have to work hard often day, evenings and weekends.

It was all up to me now.

Looking back on those years, the first five years as a consultant were exhilarating.

They were exhausting too but wholly satisfying, just as I remember my first years as a junior doctor had been…

***

After qualifying in medicine at University College London in 1975 and with my house jobs completed, I was working at Basingstoke District Hospital as a senior house officer in the Accident and Emergency Department. There were just four of us with a single consultant supervising and teaching us. We worked 42 hours first-on-call and another additional 42 hours second-on-call every week. It was the first time in my medical life that I was truly on my own treating patients and it was extraordinarily exciting.

Sometimes the tasks were simple, like stitching up a minor wound or putting a greenstick wrist fracture in a back-slab plaster. At other times it was harder, when resuscitating a patient smashed up in a road traffic accident down one of Hampshire's lanes. Suddenly the crash room would be swarming with doctors and nurses as I called for help. Anaesthetists would intubate and ventilate semi-conscious patients. Medical registrars would shock others in cardiac arrest and surgeons would cart off an occasional one to theatre with a ruptured spleen. During all this mayhem nurses would be caring for frantic relatives. Blood would be flowing into large cannulas in big arm and leg veins and ventilators would be noisily pumping high concentration of oxygen into lungs.

The patients would live or die. If they died, they were transferred to the morgue and if they lived, they went to the Intensive Care Unit.

An attempted overdose in a distressed teenager would need a stomach pumped out and, after they had come to their senses, a psychiatrist called.

A drunk would lurch in abusively from the centre of town.

There was never a dull moment.

Eventually there would be a long lull and time to have a coffee before the next patient was wheeled in.

During my six months in Accident & Emergency I saw three thousand four hundred patients and made decisions on all of them.

It was a rapid learning curve.

But I made many mistakes.

One day a young man came in with pain which sounded like renal colic. He held up a piece of gravel which looked like something from a driveway. I ordered a shot of pethidine for his pain. I did not spot that he was actually an addict and had run out of his weekend supply of morphine. What I should have known is that patients with urinary stones never come into casualty stone in hand.

Another time a rather precious middle-aged gentleman came in with abdominal pain. When I asked him to remove his clothes so that I might examine him, he was oddly reticent to oblige me. I enlisted the help of the senior sister in the department who helped remove his clothes. To my amazement he was wearing a pair of Marks & Spencer best black lace knickers and bra. My embarrassment was greater than his as I confirmed that he did not have an acute abdominal problem.

Like most doctors, I quickly learnt that this was a minor aberration compared with those patients that really like to push the boat out, such as the gentleman with a still-trembling vibrator stuck up his rectum. He said his wife had been pleasuring him but had lost her grip. It took a general anaesthetic and some nifty hand-work with grasping forceps by the surgical registrar to retrieve the apparatus and give it back to its embarrassed owner.

As a young doctor I learnt bit by bit that there is nothing stranger than folk.

Much more recently a young Chinese man with a pain in his anus was found to have a light bulb stuck the wrong way up his nether region. I was proposing to rescue the apparatus surgically when a manager interfered. It was at the time that there was a lot of press coverage concerning foreigners coming over to the UK for free medical treatment.

'Mr. McDonald, this man is not entitled to NHS treatment as he is not resident in Britain,' the manager said officiously.

'But he has a light bulb stuck in his rectum. I would classify that as an emergency! Wouldn't you?'

'He is not eligible and he has no travel insurance to pay for it privately either,' the manager continued.

There then followed a discussion through an interpreter about how the man might pay for it if we removed it for him. He shook his head a lot and said 'Ah so!' several times. After ten minutes he slipped his clothes on and said something like 'Heathrow' and 'going back to China.' A minute later he was gone into the night.

Another time in casualty I was incising a large, red, swollen abscess on a cheek. I knew it was filled with pus and I was looking forward to relieving the patient of her pain. I injected local anaesthetic liberally into it and went off to have a cup of tea while it slowly numbed the area. This minor operation was right at the limit of my surgical prowess at the time so I was quite nervous.

When I am nervous, I do one of two things. Either I talk too much or I hold my mouth open a short way and stick out my tongue and rotate it in a kind of gyrating movement. Christina has often commented unfavourably on this frog-like behaviour.

The policy of the consultant-in-charge of the Accident & Emergency at Basingstoke was that masks were a waste of time and money. There has long been argument about the efficacy of masks as witnessed by the recent debates in the Covid-19 era. Until recently even some surgical theatres eschewed their use. Indeed, they were nowhere to be found in the department at Basingstoke in those far-off days.

I scrubbed up, ready to incise the abscess, and checked the field of surgery which I was glad to find completely numb. I plucked up enough courage and I plunged a number-11 blade sharply into the abscess. Success. A spurt of yellow pus under pressure shot upwards towards the ceiling.

Unfortunately, I was directly in line with the trajectory of this fountain of white blood cells. Mouth wide open with tongue gyrating, the pus went straight down the back of my throat, coating the region of my pharynx where my tonsils once were.

It was a mistake I would never make again.

***

After six months it was time to move on to my first senior house officer post in general surgery. My work at Basingstoke had convinced me that I wanted to be a surgeon and not a psychiatrist or a gynaecologist. I had secured a post in Barnet General Hospital in North London which is not very far from where I now work in Harrow.

This small district hospital was a great place to carry out my first operations. I was supervised by a registrar at weekends but during the weekday nights I was flying solo with only a consultant on the telephone at home. It was scary at first as I was often working at the limit of my ability. I learnt quickly to make my own decisions and call for help only when needed. After calling in the consultant to help me dislodge a stuck appendix a couple of times, I learnt enough tricks to enable me to get the troublesome organ out on my own from then on.

One day, an old surgeon doing a locum in his seventies taught me that I could close the layers of the abdominal wall with catgut dissolvable stitches just as he had been taught fifty years before by a famous surgeon called Hamilton Bailey. I knew this was a bit old-fashioned as by 1976 most surgeons were using stronger non-dissolvable sutures for greater security. As predicted after removing a filthy, black appendix one night and closing the abdominal wound by his method, I watched it fall apart a week later. I realised then I would have to use more modern materials. As they say: 'Good judgement comes from bad judgement'.

As time went on my surgical repertoire expanded. One night I admitted a woman with a strangulated femoral hernia. She had been vomiting for twenty-four hours and had noticed a painful lump in her groin. This contained a knuckle of small bowel. Irreducible and obstructed, it was probably losing its blood supply too. Hence the terrible sounding term we use for this phenomenon: strangulated. It was two o'clock in the morning and I took her to theatre with the chapter in Rob & Smith's Operative Surgery open on the diathermy machine to guide me.

I followed the procedure to the letter but got a bit confused when I found an unexpected muscle in my path. I cut into it and what appeared to be urine in large quantity flowed out into the wound I had made. I panicked and took off my gown and gloves and called the consultant at home in bed. I was sure he would not welcome the call when I told him what had happened. Luckily for me it was the gentlest of the four consultants in the hospital who was on-call that night. I had feared it might be the chain-smoking, bad-tempered one who always shouted at everyone.

His voice was very reassuring on the phone. He listened for a minute and said:

'Peter, don't worry. Everything will be OK. We've all entered the bladder by mistake at one time or another. Just put a catheter in and sew up the bladder wall if you can. But do not worry because it will mend itself just by having the tube in for a couple of weeks. Next time I would advise putting a catheter in before you start an emergency femoral hernia.'

Gently admonished I put a catheter in, sewed up the bladder and closed the wound and went to bed. The consultant was right. Apart from the patient having to have a tube in her bladder for ten days after she went home, she was fine. It was a close shave and another good lesson learnt.

As the months in Barnet wore on, I was hard studying anatomy and physiology in my spare time for the dreaded Royal College of Surgeons Part I examination. With only a quarter of candidates passing first time it was an important obstacle and one I wanted to complete soon. I was planning my next foreign adventure and I hoped it would be in the bag before that. I was lucky. After attaching myself to the anatomy department of my old medical school and doing some part-time anatomy dissection, I took the examination at the first opportunity and, slightly to my amazement, I sailed through. This first hurdle was completed painlessly but the next hurdle in the form of the final FRCS examination would be a different matter.

But that is another story.

Having overcome this first hindrance to my future as a surgeon, I could indulge myself in my next unconventional escapade.

It was to become an expedition doctor.

***

Sometime during the long, hard year as a houseman, I had placed an advertisement in a magazine called Expedition.

Young doctor, 24, is looking for an expedition to join as medical officer. Anything interesting considered.

To my astonishment I had about ten calls asking me to consider their expeditions. From the British Antarctic Survey to a team going into the Highlands of Borneo, it was clear there was a shortage of adventurous medics wanting to be expedition doctors.

In among these offers, there was one from the Carlisle Mountaineering Club that looked promising. A man called Stuart Hepburn called me from Cumbria. He had a border accent and sounded interesting.

'Have you ever done any mountaineering before Peter?' he asked.

'A bit of rock climbing as a youth. But I am a keen hill-walker,' I replied.

'Well, we're hoping to drive overland to the Indian Kishtwar Himalaya and bag a couple of unclimbed peaks while we're there. If you wanted to come along as our medic, we could teach you snow and ice climbing over the next eighteen months. Interested?'

This sounded better than interesting so I agreed to learn more about their plans. He met me a week later in London on a floating restaurant moored at the Victoria Embankment alongside the Thames. I liked Stuart's vision for the trek instantly. His organised approach and his fund-raising ability confirmed he was a good man to have as leader of the expedition. It was the beginning of a friendship which has continued to this day. Over the ensuing two years the ten-man team had a dozen training meetings in the English Lake District and in Scotland.

A week's winter climbing on the north face of Ben Nevis from a hut at the head of the Alt a'Mhuilinn was the coldest week of my life. Another weekend entailed digging a snow hole and sleeping within it only to find that by the end of the night the snow ceiling had collapsed and was touching the end of my nose. As I suffer from more than a touch of claustrophobia, it was not an exercise I wanted to repeat. Slowly after many weekends climbing in the Lake District, I learnt the basics, enough to allow me to avoid being a burden to the team when in the mountains.

My task was to educate the group as to the risks of altitude and the sickness that comes with ascending too quickly into the thin air of the high peaks. I had learnt that on one of the mountains we were to climb, Sickle Moon (6,470 metres / 21,570 feet), the oxygen saturation would be just 70% of the sea level concentration. This would result in a more rapid pulse and respiration with a shift of fluid from the circulation into the cells. The team would experience breathlessness, nausea, appetite loss, vomiting, headache and extreme fatigue.

These physiological changes are more severe by sleeping high on the mountain before acclimatisation has occurred. The resultant pulmonary oedema (fluid build-up in the lungs) and cerebral oedema (swelling of the brain) can lead to respiratory failure and coma. The key to preventing these problems is to ascend no more than 500 metres per day and descend immediately if symptoms appear.

The second problem of high mountains is the cold from the altitude and high winds leading to wind-chill and frostbite. Not much adaptation to cold occurs in humans so I emphasised the need to protect hands, feet and faces at all times.

We would be at least seven days from medical help when in the high mountains and I had to be prepared for any medical eventuality. I had examined all the team and made sure they were fully protected by vaccinations and did not have any underlying health problems. I assembled 45kg of medical supplies which I hoped I would never have to use. I waited for the journey to start but, as I had done the overland route to India six years before using public transport by train, boat and bus, I knew what to expect.

In August 1977 half the team of ten climbers, including me, drove off in two donated British Leyland Sherpa vans while the remainder flew out to Delhi three weeks later. Although not a sturdy vehicle like a Land Rover, these tinny but roomy motors performed remarkably well over the bumpy roads of Europe, Turkey, Iran and Afghanistan. We motored happily over the Khyber Pass to Pakistan and then into India. There were a few adventures on the way but compared with today's political landscape these countries were peaceful and quite charming places to travel through in those days. Since the Islamic Revolution in Iran, the Russian and then the NATO invasion of Afghanistan and the Taliban-inspired instability in Pakistan, these lands are seen as too unsafe to journey through today. A sad indictment of well- or ill-intentioned interference from all points of the geographical compass.

Even the disputed Vale of Kashmir was moderately tranquil in 1977. The spruce, silver fir, birch and juniper trees growing high in the mountains made us think of the Alps but the ubiquitous marijuana plant gave it an added pungency. Populated by subsistence tenant farmers, most made a living tending crops or grazing a few lean animals. Tuberculosis, malnutrition, intestinal parasites, typhoid and rheumatic fever still afflicted the inhabitants of these high plateaus and deep valleys. As we moved higher, we saw traces of Himalayan bears and heard the shrill calls of marmots. A few snow leopards, eagles and ibex herds live in the mountains of the remote Kishtwar area bordering on China. It is also home to the nomadic herders, the Gujar and the Bukarwal. This region is just south of the area of Ladakh disputed by China and India which is today a zone of dangerous tension between the two most populous countries on earth.

By now we had parked the vans and were making our way up the valleys aided by thirty-two ponies each carrying 44kg loads. We bought provisions, met our official liaison officer, Farid, and began our trek into the high Himalaya. A four-day walk brought us to Kiar at the entrance to the upper valley of Sarbal, where we would set up Base Camp at 12,000ft.

At Kiar I got to work. News that there was a doctor in the team had preceded our entry into the village. Until that moment apart from a knee effusion and a few fleas caught at Abdullah's Tea Stall, I had hardly been consulted by the climbing team so I felt somewhat redundant. But here was a queue waiting for me in the village square. It appeared as busy as an outpatient department at home. I handed out medicines for worms, vitamin pills for malnutrition, antacids and antidiarrhoeals.

On the surgical side there was a laceration on a hand to sew up and a fractured skull in a woman with a nasty scalp wound that needed stitching. My operation on her head under local anaesthetic began with the patient sitting in a rickety old chair but she soon fainted and fell into the mud. Perhaps it was due to the attention she was receiving from the whole village or my poor attempt at anaesthesia? However, I completed the surgery, bandaged her, and got someone to carry her home. When we later returned six weeks later after the climb, she was fit and well and the first to greet us in the village square.

We marched on up the valley the next day and were now high in the mountains. We began the climb and started the setting up of the high camps. Altitude symptoms began to be felt with varying intensity by members of the team. I noted irritability, slowness in decision-making and several headaches.

One climber suffered from snow blindness while another sustained an anterior dislocation of his right shoulder after a fall at 14,000ft. Luckily before I managed to reach him, he was supported by two members of the team for an hour which prevented him slipping further down the hill. After giving him some pethidine, I was able to reduce the shoulder and he climbed back down to Base Camp at Wakbal, where he rested for five days before he resumed his role as a support climber on Sickle Moon.

A dental abscess at 15,600ft forced one climber down to receive heavy analgesia. Three others developed frostbite after climbing for some hours in three feet of snow but no-one lost parts of toes or fingers after they had been rewarmed. No climber had to make an urgent descent for altitude sickness and no member of the team had need of the emergency bottle of oxygen that I had brought all the way from England.

Although Sickle Moon defeated the climbers allocated to it, as the expedition doctor, I was spared any major medical problems. We were, in fact, the first expedition to climb that mountain without a fatality or serious injury.

This good luck allowed me to concentrate on my newly acquired climbing skills. With three others I was tasked to climb the unnamed peak on the other side of the valley. Roy, one of the climbers, got separated from the party one evening and was marooned by a thirty foot wide channel of meltwater that had rapidly appeared. It was dark and there was no alternative but to throw him a rope and let him take his chances. He moved into the waist-deep freezing water. When it reached chest height, he almost lost his balance. He finally reached us and I frog-marched him back to the advanced base camp, pulled off his soaked clothes and put him in a sleeping bag with a tot of whisky and a hot soup.

He was fine by the morning.

We began our climb to the summit of the unnamed peak, 6,392 metres (20,970ft). With, by now, only three of us fit for the climb we bivouacked at 15,000ft, and the next night at 17,500ft. The next morning, we forced on our frozen boots and cramponned up a steep snow slope for which we needed a fixed rope. Our final night before the summit push was at 19,000ft.

That night we ate a few bars of chocolate and had a brew of weak tea. I was suffering badly from the altitude with a fearful headache. I did not sleep at all. It was a miserable night with ice forming on the inside of our tent. To make matters worse the ice would break off and fall onto our faces and sleeping bags.

Next morning after a brief vomit I felt a little better. It was time to press on. We should have started climbing earlier in the morning considering avalanches become much more frequent as the sun bears down on the slopes. At 9.30am we began the final climb lethargically, squinting in the brilliant sunshine. We reach the high point from the day before after an hour and a half and sat down for a rest. One of the climbers, Roger, went ahead a few paces when I heard a shout.

'Christ I'm away!'

I saw him sliding down the slope on the edge of a huge wind slab avalanche that he had unwittingly started. He danced frantically back across the moving snow to us and threw himself on his ice-axe. The snow rumbled past and fell 3,000ft onto the glacier below. Dazed and suddenly awakened from our fatigued, quasi-meditative state, we considered the situation. Should we continue or should we turn back? I felt too unwell to contribute usefully to the discussion. Finally, two of us, Roger and I, decided to descend and we reached the safety of Camp One seven hours later.

Roy suffering from an infected finger took a risk and pressed on alone. This chain-smoker was the least fit but perhaps the most determined member of the whole team. He slowly climbed to the crest of the ridge above and trod a delicate course between its corniced edge and the break point of the avalanche. Over a false summit and across an intervening col he found himself confronted by another avalanche which broke from the summit snowfield. But Roy managed to step sufficiently clear of the sliding snow not to be troubled by it.

He plodded up the final slope and at 2.30pm on the 7th October 1977 reached the summit of the unnamed peak. He stood there for forty-five minutes gazing across the ocean of white crested Himalayan Peaks stretching far into Pakistan, Tibet and Nepal. To the south he could see the still undefeated Sickle Moon. His summit still-life photo of his ice-axe, red beret and packet of Gold Flake cigarettes was testament to his quirkiness and his resolve.

But Roy needed to move fast. It was late in the day and the descent was full of potential hazards. It would be five hours before he reached the comfort and safety of Camp One. He passed the ledge at our second bivouac where we had left him a tent in case he had need of it that night. Although it was late in the day and the light would be fading soon, he dismantled the tent and collected the items we had left for him. He continued the arduous descent rapidly and spotted us two hours ahead descending a steep snow gully. Down over the buttress and the broken ground and he arrived at Camp One an hour after dusk safe but victorious.

We revelled in his triumph reflecting that, if all three of us had tried for the summit, our combined weight might have started another and much bigger avalanche. Perhaps one man risking it alone had been the best decision. It was Roy's birthday and the peak became officially known as Janam meaning birth in Urdu. After a long rest the next afternoon we lugged all the equipment from Camp One back to Wakbal where we washed, rested and ate heartily. Roy's finger was still bad and he was now affected by snow blindness and was forced to rest in his tent away from sunlight. The next day we walked back down to Base Camp under the beautiful rock peak called The Cathedral. As we were greeted by the other members of the team, we took our last glimpse of Janam above us.

We said goodbye to it without regret.

It had been a capricious friend.

Reunited with the rest of the team we prepared for the seventy mile walk back to Kishtwar which would take five days. From that point the five who had flown out to India drove off in the Sherpa vans while we headed to Delhi to catch a flight to London.

It had been a rewarding experience being an expedition doctor and back in England I commenced a lecture tour of universities and women's institutes with an illustrated talk on Mountain Medicine. An article in Geographical magazine clumsily sub-edited and given the terrible title 'Top People Get Headaches' added to my slight notoriety.

This adventure sabbatical that I had taken during my training as a surgeon was now over. It was a good break that refreshed my batteries before I threw myself back into the task of gaining more surgical experience.

Not long after I found myself working as a Senior House Officer in Northampton General Hospital, which boasted the longest corridor in the NHS. I was back again at the coalface of British surgery ready for the cut and thrust which would lead, a dozen years later, to Northwick Park Hospital in Harrow.

Chapter 6:
A Consultant Job Brings Tricky Patients

❖

It was June 1991, and I had achieved my goal of working as a consultant surgeon in the National Health Service. I was now at Northwick Park Hospital in Northwest London. Living away from home during weekdays in the first few months was hard for both Christina and me when there was a new born baby and other children at home to be cuddled and cared for. After a long day, I would slink back sulkily to my rented room in the hospital, do some paperwork, read, relax, and sleep to be ready for the next day.

Occasionally, I would look at the local newspapers and scan the estate agents for houses to rent and wonder if they would suit Christina and the growing number of children. Despite having plenty to think about at work I missed the family dreadfully. Although I had left my parents' home and headed to Africa soon after my eighteenth birthday I had, somewhat to my surprise, become quite a doting husband and father in just a handful of years. Certainly, that summer during those long weekends on duty every fourth week, I found this separation particularly hard.

As a junior doctor I would have escaped to the junior doctors' mess for company. But in recent years the sparkle of hospital mess-life for medical staff in the NHS has begun to fade. Doctors are marrying younger so many leave the hospital to go home the moment their duties are complete. The concept that the hospital dominates your life as it did in former times is rapidly disappearing. The result is that fewer staff frequent the mess.

Formerly, it was a refuge where at any time of the day or the night you could swap a few pleasantries and gossip with a colleague from another service. Much important information about patients was shared in the mess and quick referrals and requests to give an opinion about a patient's problems were made. This was useful from the clinical care aspect and facilitated urgent care changes.

I remembered how, when I was a junior doctor, I had been irritated by the occasional over-familiar consultant who would come into the mess uninvited and read the newspapers that we had paid for. The presence of a consultant inhibited the natural gossip of the group often resulting in an awkward silence.

I remembered what one of my friends had told me when he became a consultant in Suffolk. Once every six months the consultants in his department treated the junior staff to a slap-up meal in a local Chinese restaurant. It was always a very jolly affair and plenty of alcohol was drunk. I suppose today it would be called team building.

'That must have been great for morale!' I applauded. 'I will try and do the same when I become a consultant. I bet you had some great evenings.'

'Yes, we did Peter but we consultants always went home early.'

'Oh! And why was that?'

'Because the juniors could not wait for us all to leave so that they could really let their hair down.'

Such is the nature of hierarchy. Medical, military, academic, commercial, political. It is all much the same despite the first name calling that is present in some organisations with the faux camaraderie disguising it. In the NHS it is changing too but the day I became a consultant in 1991 was the day that only other consultants called me by my given name. I was 'mister' or 'sir' from that day forward for the rest.

Perhaps I had assumed the consultants' common room would be a substitute for the junior doctors' mess and that I would hardly miss it. In this assumption I was proved very wrong. Not only was the consultants' common room at Northwick Park cold and uninviting, but there was hardly ever a soul within it. During the weekdays the work patterns in a hospital revolve around the consultants so that, with only a few exceptions, their days are busy, packed with ward rounds, theatre lists, outpatient sessions, teaching, and administrative seminars.

If there was ever a chance to snatch more than just a sandwich at lunchtime it might be taken back to the consultants' common room where, at most, half a dozen colleagues would be present. I was struck just how negative the conversation was. There was much talk of the managers and administrators and their unworkable schemes. There was discussion about the mechanism of taking early retirement and plenty of imaginary reflections as to how working in the NHS was much better in the past than it was today. There were plenty of complaints concerning car parking charges and the unfairness of the clinical excellence award scheme that allows consultants to increase their remuneration from the hospital.

I was quite shocked by just how pessimistic these men and women were. I doubted that they were a representative sample of the consultant body. More a group of disaffected lunchtime moaners who maybe had not quite enough to do. Yet these were physicians and surgeons and others who had made it good in every sense. They had security, high incomes and a background of considerable attainment to be proud of. Yet here they were often behaving like five-year olds whining over chocolate fingers at a party.

Amongst them, I noticed a close colleague I had met several times before. A man only a year or two older, he had been at Northwick for ten years as a trainee and then a couple as a consultant. It was clear to me that he was a man who would be cheerless whatever fortune might bring. Whenever I offered a light-hearted good-morning, I would be greeted by a long face and a grunt which would be quickly followed by some comment suggesting how stressed he was about everything and nothing in particular.

I have long since discovered that some individuals are cheery even when sad and others appear miserable when quite happy but this colleague's feelings were clearly written on his face. He was often miserable. Around him there was an aura of discontentment that permeated down to his staff and his patients.

He seemed so stressed by so much and so little.

If ever a job required sharpness and decision-making it is being a consultant. The art of medicine is hard to master and uncertainty is part of that territory. Doctors have to get used to this. I had been well trained to think this way and so presumably had he. Yet he agonised over everything. When a patient had need of being taken to theatre immediately, he would prevaricate by ordering further tests. If another needed more time before it was clear as to what was required, he would worry himself silly by visiting the patient again and again until both patient and doctor were weary. Just occasionally this stress would express itself in the form of a brusque response to a patient. When there was a crowd in outpatients, he would sometimes lose his temper and a patient would get the raw end of his tongue.

I have learnt painfully over the years that I cannot be liked by all my patients but direct complaints about my manner are quite rare for I am a cheery kind of soul. However, occasionally a joke misfires when I am trying to inject humour into my clinical practice in order to lighten the load for a patient. When that happens a complaint can follow, suggesting I was offhand or unprofessional. In the modern era, which has been described as the era when deference has collapsed, health professionals will hear quickly of their shortcomings from their patients through the complaints procedures now available to the patients. Strangely these criticisms, often destructive, spurious or simple misunderstandings, are actively encouraged by hospitals. There are even signs up in the corridors telling patients how to make their grievances known to managers or, worse still, to lawyers.

Although this colleague was in fact a very competent doctor despite his mental anguish, he did create a small stream of refugees from his clinics. Some would find their way via their GPs to my outpatient clinic and I would have to try and pick up the pieces.

***

One such patient was Winifred Granger. She had originally been referred to my colleague's clinic with constipation and a change in bowel habit. As she was of advancing years her GP had wisely arranged for her to have a barium enema. Nowadays we would perform a CT colonogram or a colonoscopy but this was still the heyday of the sticky white barium. Winifred had undergone one a few years previously so she knew what was expected. Purgation followed by insufflation of barium and air up the rectum and then being twiddled around under an X-ray machine.

Winifred's colon was revealed as capacious but structurally normal. As the GP was still unable to get his patient's bowels working properly, he referred her to the hospital.

'When I told Dr. Smith that I could not go to the toilet in the mornings without an enema he was not really interested. He seemed to be preoccupied with something else and I am not sure he took much notice of me. All he said was that I was OK and that I was lucky not to have cancer and that I must cope as best I can.'

'Well, Mrs. Granger that was good reassuring advice I think,' I replied.

'But I really cannot go unless I sit on the toilet for hours each morning, Mr. McDonald. And I have to strain terribly!'

'Do you feel ill with it?' I asked.

'No not ill. Just not right. Anyway, it cannot be right to have all that pooh inside, can it?'

'Constipation has never been shown to do any harm though, Mrs. Granger,' I soothed.

'Well, it's not right so I have to get it out one way or another with a finger!' she continued.

'Some of my patients need to do that. It is something I hear quite often. Let me prescribe some stronger purgative to help you be more regular. I would also like to refer you to our Biofeedback team to see if they can ease the problem for you.'

'Oh yes, Mr. McDonald that would be nice,' she agreed.

Over the course of the next six months Mrs. Granger paid four visits to the Biofeedback Department. These therapists enthusiastically specialise in trying to retrain patients in order for them to cope with their real or perceived defaecatory disorders. In a world where the biggest selling therapies in the world are purgatives, stool softeners, suppositories and enemas, there is no shortage of patients wanting their help. With great diligence they take these 'worried well' patients through the ritual of passing stool. Squatting, abdominal pressure, relaxation and dietary advice all form part of it.

Despite its unglamorous nature the worry that constipation, or obstructed defaecation, causes is out of all proportion to its medical importance to the patient. For most of us toileting is second nature. However, for Mrs. Granger and millions of others it becomes the overriding concern of the day. It may dominate their conversation, thinking and even their social life.

With this in mind, it was not surprising that when I reviewed Mrs. Granger after a further six months, she was still an unhappy soul.

'I am not much better Mr. McDonald, you know. The Biofeedback team were very nice but I still cannot go. It is not right. No. It is not right at all!'

'Mrs. Granger, let me reassure you that you are not alone in all this. A third of the population are unhappy about their bowels. Half the world complain that they pass unnatural amounts of wind and, unfortunately, their partners collude with them by agreeing that this wind must be abnormal. Others have to strain to get the job done. But this problem for you will not worsen and it will not harm you.'

'But can't you operate and make it better, Mr. McDonald?'

'Well, actually Mrs. Granger I do not advise that.' I retorted.

In the early part of the twentieth century Mrs. Granger, if she had independent means, might have had her way. William Arbuthnot Lane, a London surgeon, had attributed all manner of ailments to the colon and had removed it as often as possible. Sub-total colectomy, as it was called, had become quite the fashion.

However, it became quite clear that many more problems followed such radical treatment than pre-existed before the operation. Colectomy, or removal of all or part of the colon, has largely been abandoned for anything other than cancer or severe inflammation of the colon from colitis or diverticulitis. Few surgeons would today advocate surgery for severe constipation unless the colon was grossly dilated. I have only performed one such intervention in thirty years and it was not a great success. However, a colostomy, or a simple stoma, to relieve the symptoms may very occasionally be indicated.

Winifred's colon was structurally and physiologically normal so was best left in place.

'No. I do not think it would be a good idea for you to have a colectomy Mrs. Granger,' I continued.

'You mean I just have to carry on as now?'

'Mrs. Granger, a surgeon like me, knows when he is powerless to help. I am afraid your case is one that would not benefit from surgery. It would make everything a lot harder for you, actually. Much as I would like to wave a magic wand and make you instantly better I cannot. But I know I can make you a lot worse than you are now if I offered you an operation.'

'So, I will have to live with this constipation for the rest of my life?'

'Yes, but it usually does not get deteriorate further and I think you will be all right in the long run.'

She looked crestfallen and was silent for a moment until she added tearfully.

'As long as I can come up and see you from time to time, I suppose I will manage?'

'That would be fine, Mrs. Granger. That is what I am here for. Not always to operate but often to reassure.'

That last exchange is telling. It illustrates how surgeons are not just technicians but must be good doctors too. As Theodor Kocher, the great Swiss surgeon and the father of thyroid surgery, wrote: 'A surgeon is a man who knows how to operate but must know when not to.'

This simple sentence should be understood by managers and administrators who count costly operations and outpatient visits like beans. They need to appreciate that patients may require to be reassured by repeated visits and not operations. Indeed, this kind of care is a lot cheaper than performing inappropriate surgery.

All the patient may need is someone in clinic who understands them and who can talk through their problem however banal their difficulties are. Not all patients can be instantly discharged with the 'consultant episode' completed and the cost charged to whoever has commissioned it. GPs know this more than most. It is a lesson often forgotten in the rush to get patients processed by the system as if they were widgets being manufactured and sold by the kilogram.

Although Mrs. Granger left my clinic that day disappointed, she was not unhappy. I knew she would continue to cope with her miserable, unmentionable condition and that I would have to give a little of my time every now and then to help her. Some doctors find this sort of patient irritating but much of the job of being a good clinician is doing just that.

Reassuring.

Smiling.

Cajoling.

Caring.

As a surgeon my serious complication rate after major intestinal operations is about five per cent, which is about average for my type of high risk surgery. But my serious complication rate when I do not operate is an impressive zero per cent. Not bad eh?

As I was steadily learning this lesson of medical reassurance, I realised there were a lot of patients in my colorectal practice that I could not help. Those with irritable bowel syndrome, constipation, obstructed defecation, non-specific abdominal pain and the like. All branches of medicine have similar patients and although some doctors have termed them 'heartsink' or 'functional problem' patients these are not really very helpful concepts. These labels are not very respectful to the patients suffering from these syndromes which conventional medicine cannot cure.

There is a pressing need to find alternatives to the allopathic medicine that conventional doctors practise. This search for other lines of treatment is more likely to occur if the patients have a poor rapport with the specialist or GP. What patients hate most is being patronised by a doctor who has no idea as to why they have their symptoms and even less understanding as to how to treat them. Whichever branch of medicine we practice, we get used to this feeling of inadequacy and just learn to help our patients cope.

My rules are quite simple.

Tell the patient that they do not suffer alone and that there are many others like them.

Try to understand them.
Never blame the patient because you don't know what the cure is.

***

Every day when I used to wake my children up in the mornings to go to school, I used to say to them before I rushed out of the house: 'Be good, be kind, be happy!'

It irritated them beyond measure but should it not be a lesson for doctors in training on a daily basis too?

But we need to train those in healthcare management the same philosophy. Counting operations on a spreadsheet may help cash flow but it is only a small part of the medicine.

We will see shortly what happens when only numbers of operations are counted and when no consideration is taken of quality.

Chapter 7: How Management Makes Matters Worse

❖

Since 1949, when the NHS was founded, it has been perpetually trying to reinvent itself. Like cricket in the rain, it is a kind of national obsession.

Since the so-called reforms of the NHS in the late 1980s the top person in a hospital has been the Chief Executive. In order for everyone to know that there was a true break from the past the government even changed the name of the places the doctors and nurses worked in. Suddenly our workplaces were transformed from hospitals – hospitalia in Latin, meaning an apartment for strangers or guests – to 'trusts', deriving from Middle English, meaning confident, safe, secure. Reassuring perhaps for English-speaking Anglo-Saxons finally vanquishing our Roman conquerors but all rather confusing if you ask me.

I have always regarded organisational name changing for its own sake rather a childish exercise. We have learnt over the years that politicians, by their very nature, need to alter things whether they are broken or not. Each time they are elected they must be seen to have made their mark. This is their modus operandi. Changing names is the cheapest way of expressing this need, much like a tomcat sprays his territory.

The fact that these changes make no difference to the working efficiency of an institution is strangely overlooked. The excitement of seeing official letterheads and logos transformed is too great a temptation for administrators and managers.

Just before the new wave of NHS reforms were introduced in the late 1980s an influential report chaired by the head of a supermarket chain stated that it would be a good idea to bring in outsiders and put them in charge. After all, if the doctors could not be trusted and the hospital administrators were ineffectual, why not bring in executives from high street chains or retired military men and see if they could do a better job?

So it was that ex-Rear Admiral Michael Cole had been appointed Chief Executive of the new Northwick Park Hospital Trust. It was said that he had been effective in his role in the Navy and was noted to be quite the diplomat. It therefore seemed quite appropriate for him to take his retirement pension from the Navy and try his hand in another post where his ample organisational skills might be used to good effect.

When he visited the fifty-five-acre sprawling site in Harrow for the first time he was a bit shocked by what he found. A hospital that was not more than twenty years old that looked like something from a horror movie. In fact, Northwick Park had been used in a famous film in that genre, Alien. This speaks volumes for its aesthetic qualities.

As Michael Cole looked deeper into Northwick's functioning, he could see the deep-seated problems of organisation that he was confident he could sort. Although he had never had any contact with medicine apart from ordering around a few oft-inebriated surgeon commanders in the Navy, he did not let that lack of experience worry him. It should not be too hard to learn the ropes on the job? After all, government ministers shift from portfolio to portfolio on the whim of a Prime Minister's reshuffle, so why would not he?

At his own interview ex-Admiral Michael Cole's smooth charm, fine features, warm smile and fluent answers had so impressed the committee that they unanimously gave him the job over others many of whom had worked rather too long in the NHS to be trusted. Four weeks later Michael was installed in his spacious office overlooking the front entrance to the hospital. From his window he could admire the newly painted sign Northwick Park Hospital Trust and was pleased to see his own name as Chief Executive printed in bold letters underneath. At least everyone knew now who was in charge.

One of his first duties was to meet all the newly appointed consultants and, as my interview had been the first he had officiated at, he began with me in my tiny office with that view of Harrow School. He tapped on my door one lunchtime a few weeks after I had started.

'How are you settling in Mr. McDonald? Or can I call you Peter?'

'Of course. Yes. Nicely thank you, Michael. I seem to have everything in place to allow me to get on with the task. Good colleagues, a first-class secretary and a neat little office. Yes, I can say I am truly enjoying it and I hope to make my mark here.'

'Good, to hear it, Peter. Certainly, your senior colleague has indicated that you have made a good start. If there is anything else you need please come and ask anytime. I like to keep an open door for the consultants. As the cliché goes, please don't hesitate to contact me.'

'Thank you Michael I will bear that in mind,' I said looking at my watch.

'Time I got to theatre.'

'Er, before you go to theatre, Peter, I wanted to tell you about my new waiting list initiative. I am hoping to have the cooperation of all the surgical staff to get all the long-waiters operated on in the next three months so that the Trust can benefit from the incentive scheme arrangements just announced by the Regional Health Authority. What we plan to do is to fix a date for all patients who have waited more than eighteen months. What do you think, Peter?'

I had been involved peripherally in waiting list initiatives in several of my training posts. They had usually been feeble gestures and had often failed to achieve their aims. At the same time, they had severely disrupted the working routines of the hospital. It was not that I did not want to help, because the scandal of the British NHS is its lack of access for its patients. Seeing a GP, being referred to a consultant, accessing investigations, and getting an operation or a treatment takes far too long. Until there is a real incentive to create a consumer-style experience by allowing the wages of those doing it to be linked directly to their activity, I cannot ever see it succeeding.

As I write this I think of my step-son Oliver in Australia who pays a modest fee to the Queensland State Health system. Less than £750 per annum. When a calculus got stuck in his right ureter due to the heat of the Queensland sun, it blocked his right kidney, causing him excruciating pain. One phone call and he was able to see his GP in two hours. A scan was arranged that morning in a nearby privately run facility and a urologist saw him the same afternoon and gave him sound advice.

In the NHS where I work that same process would have resulted in a wait in an Accident & Emergency of several hours. Then a multiple day wait for a scan before being able to see a urologist six weeks later. The NHS is far from a perfect service even with urgent problems. When the case is routine it is even worse.

Hence the Chief Executive's quite reasonable request to expedite admission for patients who had been waiting eighteen months already.

'Will there be more operating lists and more time to get the urgent and emergency cases done as well?' I naively asked. 'My waiting times are already lengthening. It will need more theatre nurses and technicians.' I continued. 'Is the Health Authority giving us more money to do it?'

'Well, er, no, not exactly Peter. You see it is all a question of prioritising and cutting out inefficiency. Trust me, I was an admiral!', he joked.

Michael liked the sound of his own jokes and his loud jovial laugh could be heard all around the hospital. I imagined he had been the life and soul of the wardroom in all the Royal Navy ships he had sailed in.

Despite my reservations as to his plan, instinctively I liked the man.

'But Michael, it won't be easy to get the waiting lists down unless the urgent cases are catered for as well.'

'Nonsense, my boy, with slick keen young consultants like you around we cannot fail to make a difference.'

'Thanks for the flattering comment but I am not sure I quite see how?'

'Now you had better get off to your list Peter. We will talk about it another time,' he chided me.

I skipped down the stairs and headed for the theatre corridor wondering how the Chief Executive's plan would work. I could not see how his approach was practical. Was I missing some hidden ingredient in it all? I put these thoughts out of my mind and went in to change into my scrubs and start the first case.

The list which included two colon cancer resections went without incident.

***

It was not long before the waiting list initiative was put into full force. A senior manager had been co-opted from the Regional Health Authority to mastermind the Trust's efforts. She came to see me. She was rather bossy and had an unpleasant manner. I was not surprised that she was on secondment rather than having a regular job.

'I have booked the long waiters on your operation lists for the next six weeks. Gall bladders, hernias, haemorrhoids. You know the sort of thing. All left over from your predecessor's time. That will be about fifty cases. Region will be delighted as we are rolling out the programme across ENT and orthopaedics as well.'

And so, it was that the programme began, like a steamroller over the fields of Northwick Park Hospital. Organised by a manager who knew nothing about my practice and even less about the clinical cases. A manager who would listen to no suggestions or accept any modifications to her plan. After all, it was based on a format worked out by the Department of Health itself. It must be good. It would be bound to succeed.

The result was a spectacular failure.

There were even more disappointed patients than usual.

This fact is best illustrated by Alfred Williams' large irreducible hernia. He had first been seen fifteen months earlier by my predecessor. As he had suffered a severe heart attack a few months prior to being seen, putting him through the day case unit was thought to be too risky. It was decided that a spinal block would be the most appropriate method of anaesthesia.

He was therefore put on the routine list as his rupture was not too painful. On that list he waited as was the custom of the NHS. At the nine-month mark a computer registered that he was still on the list and something called a validation exercise was carried out. The computer generated a letter to Alfred asking him, on behalf of the Trust, if he still needed his hernia operation.

It came as a bit of a surprise to Alfred to be asked such a question as he was certain the hernia was still there and it hurt a lot. Just in case he was in error he dropped his pyjamas in front of his bathroom mirror and asked his wife for a second opinion. Seeing the hernia staring back at them in the mirror they both agreed that he still required the operation and so wrote back to the hospital accordingly. In consequence Alfred and his hernia were left on the waiting list.

At the fifteen-month mark, with his wife's dementia worsening, the computer indicated that he was now a red alert patient approaching the maximum tolerated waiting limit. Another office in the administrative wing of the hospital would now be asked to deal with his case. Without informing me, his name was pencilled on to my operating list with three other long waiters for an operation the next Monday. Knowing there were two urgent cancers already scheduled for that day I went to see the bossy waiting list manager again.

'There are at least four waiting list patients on my list and I am sure we will run out of time to do them as I have two cancers planned for that day as well as an emergency admission with bowel obstruction that is being worked up for operation too.'

'I think we should postpone Alfred Williams and two others as they will not get done.'

'I am sorry Mr. McDonald but we cannot cancel the patients once they are booked in. Regional policy and all that. I expect you'll find the time.'

I was more than annoyed by this manager's attitude but after protesting for a few more minutes and getting no further I went off to do a pre-operative ward round. The list in question was being scheduled and there was obviously no room for more than one long waiter so I instructed my house surgeon to put only both cancers, the bowel obstruction and one additional bilateral hernia case on the list. The latter had been cancelled once before and so had a special right to be on the list that day.

It was a nine-hour operating list and we were under clear instructions from the theatre manager and the clinical director not to overrun as the theatre staff were both exhausted and in short supply.

Later that day I got a call from the waiting list manager.

'I have just added the three long waiters to your list Mr. McDonald and we are bringing them in just in case there is time.'

I was flabbergasted at the stupidity of such an action as I was pretty sure there would not be enough time to operate on them.

'I think that is a cruel waste of time for them all. Are you going to be the one who tells them to return home without the operation after they have been starved and hospitalised?'

'Well, er, no! That's not part of my duties.'

'Well, in that case take my advice and cancel them now and stop them coming in.'

'My hands are tied Mr. McDonald. My instructions and memoranda all state that we have to follow the policy laid down by the Regional Health Authority.'

'Damn the policy!'

I slammed down the phone and continued with my paperwork. I was sure I was in the right and she was wrong.

Next Monday we got the list off to a good start although the complex anaesthesia needed for the rectal cancer patient took quite a while to establish. An epidural was administered once the patient was asleep and a urinary catheter inserted. The method of resection of a rectal cancer by any method requires a meticulous technique. It takes anything between two to five hours to do well. This time it was three-and-a-half hours but the next case was a large right sided colon tumour requiring excision and joining-up the colon to the ileum or small intestine.

It was another half hour before this case was on the table. My anaesthetist Dr. Neville Robinson, a New Zealander from Wellington, was one of the best in the business but even he was not a miracle worker. He never stops for a break and has the fastest anaesthetic hands in the hospital for putting drips up and tubes down. The case took two hours and, as there was close involvement of the right colic artery by lymph nodes, a rather more careful dissection than normal was needed.

'Ready for the obstruction case, Peter?' came Neville's encouraging Kiwi twang as he thrust open the door of the anaesthetic room with the next patient.

It was nearly half-past two and even if this case was easy it might still be difficult to fit in the bilateral hernia case let alone the other three long waiters. But our blood was up and as sometimes happens during an all-day list the team becomes more, not less, effective as the day wears on and the deadline looms.

Luckily for us that day this case was very straightforward. Through an extended incision a huge cancer of the right colon was lifted out and the two ends of the bowel stapled together in double time. The fact that the patient was obstructed made the anastomosis, or join-up, easier as the small bowel upstream was dilated to about the same size as the transverse colon lower down the gut to where it was to be sutured together.

It was now four o'clock in the afternoon and we knew we had to gallop the bilateral hernia patient on to the table to pre-empt any suggestion from the theatre manager that we should stop at that point. By five thirty with the help of my registrar operating on the other side, we had sewn the meshes in place and were closing up.

As I was writing the operating note in the surgeons' room, I remembered the other 'lost' cases. The time for operating had expired and the list was halted. They just could not be done. I knew that one of us would soon have to go to the surgical ward and tell them that we had run out of time. It was a task we all dreaded.

A thought passed through my mind.

I would get the bossy long waiting list manager to accompany me so she might see the misery she had caused. I messaged her on the long-range bleep and left a note for her to call me immediately. It was a full ten minutes before she got through. I explained the situation.

'You'll come with me to the ward to see the patients as we explain that they will have to go home without having had their operations?'

'Er, no Mr. McDonald, that's beyond my pay grade and I am already at home as I finish at 4.30pm.'

With that the line went dead. I was pretty sure she had cut me off short deliberately. Twenty minutes later I was in the surgical ward seeing the patients. I left Alfred Williams until last. The first patient, who I was not very familiar with, seemed to comprehend the situation reasonably well but the second one shouted at me. I tried to reassure them both that I would try to get them done very soon. I even told them I would endeavour to do their operations personally.

It was not the same with Alfred Williams. He did not get angry or agitated at all. After hearing me out, he just stared at the wall in front of him. He had the most despondent expression on his face that I had ever seen.

'You see, Mr. McDonald, I have had to put my wife Maud into a special respite home to cover the time of this operation. It has cost me quite a lot of money. In fact, most of my savings. I had really set my heart on having the operation today.'

I felt dreadful. This was made worse by the fact that I had known none of this.

'And, by the way, Mr. McDonald, I know it's not your fault. Perhaps I should have told you that the hernia is now beginning to hurt badly. In fact, it gets quite hard and keeps me awake at night at times.'

He rambled on a bit as he gazed at me like a man half awake.

'If I had known that it was likely my operation would be cancelled, I could have postponed Maud's admission and saved the money. We could have done it another time.'

As I heard him out it was even clearer to me then that the waiting list manager should have been present hearing this tale of woe.

I made a few phone calls to find out if there were any gaps in any of the lists in the next couple of days but they were all overbooked with urgent cases just as mine had been. Alfred went home an hour later limping a little and looking extraordinarily sad. I felt deeply upset by the whole affair and drove home in a foul mood.

Alfred Williams never got his hernia fixed on one of my main operating lists. With my growing practice there were more and more urgent and major cases with life-threatening conditions being sent to me for treatment. Patients were being referred in from all over the hospital and the region. It was only when the Regional Health Authority could see finally that we needed more lists and more staff that we were finally able to get Alfred and the other long waiters in. The managers waited until the final deadline before the end of the clinical accounting year and then threw more money at us. More theatre nurses were recruited and doctors and surgeons were employed at the weekends. It was expensive and messy and all rather rushed.

Alfred's hernia was repaired four months to the day after he had been on my list that Monday. This time it was not cancelled as he was not competing with cancers and emergencies. His recovery was unremarkable. My registrar who was by now a very competent hernia surgeon did his operation. Alfred was said to be delighted with the result even though his bank account was empty. He had, of course, had to pay for another session of respite care for Maud but this time it had not been money thrown to the wind.

The saga of Alfred's hernia was not the last time as a consultant I would witness managerial interference that made matters worse. It is not that managers do not care. Quite the reverse is the case. It is just that they are taught to ignore the experts. Experts are suspect and are seen as an untrustworthy self-interested group.

This leads administrators to create daft solutions for politically manufactured problems. You will find many more examples of this phenomenon as you turn these pages.

Chapter 8:
Georgina And Her Lover

❖

It was within a few months of starting work as a consultant at Northwick Park that I appreciated that becoming the boss, the consultant, after being a minion was a more radical change than I had anticipated.

Not only was I no longer looking over my shoulder wondering what my consultant would think, I was being asked to decide on the appointment of house officers and registrars and to give references that would influence their future careers. Although the patronage system is now considered an outdated method of determining advancement, it did have a few advantages. In return for guidance and support the patron could demand discipline and hard work from the trainee.

More importantly if the patron was caring and assiduous, they would often be a role model for those following after them. Exactly in that way forty-five years ago almost to the day, I had followed one of my consultants, Bill Heald, into the field of general surgery. He was an inspiring teacher and a remarkable surgeon who later became world famous for his work on rectal cancer. He was an inspiration and a role model though I knew I could never match his brilliance and single-minded commitment.

Today, young doctors are selected for preferment by panels of senior doctors who are permitted to ask only certain carefully selected questions. This makes the process of determining who to promote quite a sterile ritual. It is also nowhere near as enjoyable and I doubt the earnest men and women who run these parades are overwhelmed with volunteers to help them.

Of course, it is true that the old system was open to abuse.

I found this to my cost. As a registrar, I had fallen foul of an unpleasant, vindictive consultant during my training. I had displayed the temerity to criticise his behaviour both towards me and a patient in the medical press. I had written the piece as a lesson for others as to how not to behave as a consultant. The consequence was that he launched a vendetta against me. On several occasions he tried to prevent me being promoted. My advancement was certainly delayed but I battled on and finally won through in the end. In fact, just before I gained my consultant post he had the graciousness to apologise to me.

'I now realise I was wrong to try and block your promotion, Peter,' he had said after one final interview when he had sat on the panel. 'I now see you will make a good consultant surgeon. For any delay in your progression to such a post, I must apologise.'

Those two sentences from him must have cost his pride a great deal.

My personal experience of this negative patronage redoubled my resolve to help the right young trainees get along in their chosen fields. Although today we are not expected to lobby directly on their behalf in this new equal-playing-field world, I still support them in the old-fashioned ways with advice and encouragement. I will make telephone calls to future employers but those trainees I deem uncaring, lazy or ill-suited to the strenuous life in surgery, I will steer into other fields. Sloppy, unpunctual and unprofessional behaviour with staff and patients, I treat with the disdain it deserves and if the individual does not show a willingness to reform, my support for them will be withdrawn altogether.

***

Georgina Sandhurst was one of my first house surgeons.

She had been chosen from the field of thirty newly qualified doctors. As I had one of the few unlinked jobs in London, this meant that a doctor from any medical school in the land could apply. Many did, from outside and inside the capital. Georgina was bright, kind and extremely hard working. The fact that she was blonde and stunningly beautiful was a side issue which we all tried to ignore on ward rounds. However, I did note some of the young male medical staff had difficulty overlooking this fact.

Her treatment of patients was exemplary and her sensitive handling of a dying patient had been only one of many acts of compassion that I had witnessed in the few months she had worked for me. As to her own long-term aims, these were as yet undefined. At her first appraisal she had stated that, although she had enjoyed surgery, the lifestyle of a consultant surgeon with its perpetual disruptions to routine was not going to be compatible with the life outside medicine that she wanted. Perhaps she was thirty years before her time and it would be different today? At that time the profession was not as accommodating to female trainees as it should have been. It is, I hope, much more supportive today.

With regard to women in surgery, I have both enjoyed training and developing the many young women doctors who have worked for me over the years. Many have the drive, ambition and intelligence to pursue any path in medicine but are aware of the limitations that certain choices might give them. For my part I wish many more had stayed in my branch of surgery, as I know it benefits greatly from being more inclusive. Unfortunately, surgery remains a male-heavy profession although we have made steady progress in recent years and is rapidly changing.

As I write this after fifty years in medicine, I have four female surgical consultant and professorial colleagues out of twenty. Without exception these women are clever and organized and have managed to raise children and publish ground-breaking research at the same time.

No mean achievements.

Perhaps some of these thoughts were going through Georgina's mind as she worked as my house surgeon. She mentioned on a few occasions that she thought general practice or anaesthetics might fit in better with her plans. This did not stop her immersing herself in the care of our surgical patients. From the early hours to the evenings nothing was too much trouble for her. Her ability to learn quickly and her impeccable relationships with other staff shone through her work.

I have had the pleasure to have trained many very good house surgeons. As I look back over the years, she might even have been the best of the hundred or so that I have worked for me.

'I would like you to present one of our patients at Grand Rounds, Georgina,' I said to her one day.

'The patient with necrotising pancreatitis might be a good case for you. He has been with us no less than seven months and is just about to get home. His case illustrates almost all the problems a patient can suffer short of actually dying. I think our colleagues and the rest of the medical staff would be keen to hear about him.'

'Of course, Mr. McDonald. Would you like me to present a short critical review of the latest literature on the subject as well?'

'That would be most appropriate Georgina. Thanks.'

The task I was setting her was not an insubstantial one for a twenty-three year old. To present such a complex case in front of a hundred and fifty doctors in a formal lecture theatre setting is not easy. Even for this able young woman it would be a daunting prospect. A lot of work late into the night sifting through notes and reading original and highly complex papers. To crystallise all this information into a digestible and intelligible form to withstand the often-sharp criticism of the collective consultant and trainee body of Northwick Park Hospital could be a task too great for many.

However, I knew this was within Georgina's capability so when I stood up three weeks later at the opening of the Grand Round, announcing that she was to present a most interesting and complex case of 'The man who nearly died of pancreatitis', I had every confidence she would give a good account of the case and herself.

I later leant that she had wisely asked for some help from one of the senior house officers but this did not diminish my admiration for her efforts as she sailed through her slides.

Mr. J.P. aged 30 was admitted to the surgical ward on 5th September with acute pancreatitis. On admission he had shown signs of toxaemia with a tachycardia, hypotension and a white cell count of

18×10^3. He required resuscitation intravenously with five litres of normal saline, systemic broad-spectrum antibiotics and intramuscular opiates for pain relief.

Over the next 48 hours an ultrasound was carried out which confirmed gall stones but his liver function tests were only slightly deranged. A diagnosis of gall-stone pancreatitis was made and over the next three days he continued to deteriorate with a falling serum calcium. An enhanced CT scan revealed a degree of ischaemic necrosis of the body of the pancreas.

As we were unable to support him adequately on the surgical ward, he was moved to the Intensive Care Unit on the fourth day and following a further deterioration over three more days, despite full ventilation and inotropic support, Mr. McDonald carried out a, laparotomy and necrosectomy i.e. removal of all the dead pancreatic tissue.

As I sat listening to Georgina's presentation, I felt very proud on her behalf. Using the language of medicine that she had recently mastered as a student, she had succinctly explained how the patient had suffered a catastrophic inflammation of his pancreas that had led to it losing its blood supply, requiring a dangerous operation to pull out all the dead tissue. Humans only seem to be able to live with a limited amount of dying tissue before it kills them. This is certainly the case with the pancreas when it goes wrong by self-digesting itself with all the powerful enzymes that organ usually secretes to breakdown foodstuffs.

Although I was not quite old enough to be her father, marked paternal feelings were stirring within me. This young doctor was simply doing a damn fine job. She continued with the case by outlining the patient's three week stay in the ICU, the management of his infection and sepsis, his jejunostomy feeding tube placed in the second part of the small bowel and his need for extensive wound care. She highlighted several of the complications he had suffered in the months following the operation and emphasised his slow but steady progress by drawing her audience's attention to his weight chart, which after a 35% loss of gross body weight was now again within 10% of his pre-illness weight.

She followed the presentation of the case with a comprehensive review of the literature and began by acknowledging the help she had received from the senior house officer Dr. Dinesh Rao. The papers she had collated together were cleverly summarised and an overall picture of severe necrotising pancreatitis was painted for the assembled doctors. It was all very impressive for one who had never had to present to so large and well-informed an audience before.

At the conclusion of her last slide, I jumped up and thanked her warmly and said we would be happy to take questions and comments from the audience. Dr. Gary Richards, a particularly acerbic physician, was sitting in his usual place in the front row and was the first to indicate that he had a comment to make.

'Dr. Sandhurst you are to be congratulated for your presentation but do you think that all the dreadful complications and slow recovery from Mr. McDonald's operation might have been avoided if radiological drainage of the pancreas had been tried instead?'

It was Gary at his most provocative and I worried for a moment how Georgina was going to respond. It might have been better if I had fielded the question myself but I thought I would give her a moment or two to see if she might win over the audience.

'Dr. Richards that is a very interesting question indeed but I think you may have overlooked a detail in my presentation. As I mentioned the CT scan showed necrosis, or death, of three-quarters of the pancreas. The Hounsfield scores calculated from the CT scan demonstrated quite clearly that nearly all of the dead area was made up of solid components that would never be suited to external radiological drainage. Moreover, the article from the Cleveland Clinic, to which I referred, addressed this problem comprehensively and would indicate that Mr. McDonald had no alternative in a deteriorating patient than to proceed to the rarely used, but fully accepted, risky operation of pancreatic necrosectomy, crudely removing all the dead tissue.'

It was a masterly answer and, as I stood up to add a further rider to back up the science behind my decision, I was overwhelmed with admiration for young Dr. Sandhurst. A few further rather more straightforward questions were answered without difficulty and in another ten minutes the Grand Round was at an end. It was clear that Georgina was relieved it was over as she slumped in a chair and took in a large breath.

'Well done Georgina! You are a real trooper. I expect you are looking forward to your holiday next week. Where are you going by the way?'

'Australia Mr. McDonald. A distant uncle has invited me to help him with the rounding up of his four thousand sheep on his farm in the outback. It's about two hundred miles west of Sydney but it seemed a two-week break I should not miss. You know how I love horses.'

'Will you get to see the Great Barrier Reef at all? It really is fantastic,' I urged.

'No, I don't think my funds will stretch that far this time. Just enough for the flight and not many pennies more.'

***

With Georgina off on holiday, we got a student locum to do her job. He was nice but very green so we relied very much more on Dr. Dinesh Rao, the senior house officer, for the care of our ward patients. Dinesh was one of those bright, ambitious first generation British Asians. His parents had been shipped out of Uganda in a hurry when Idi Amin went bananas and Dinesh had continued his education in England. Evidently, he thrived in his new environment. He was a kindly, precise, well-spoken man who was destined to become a surgeon in the years to come. He had a grim determination to succeed at whatever he set his mind to.

With Georgina away, I was able to get a closer look at Dinesh and I liked very much what I saw. Though a pleasant looking man his looks were, at that moment in time, somewhat spoiled by a large boil on the end of his nose. Although the abscess showed signs of bursting, I tried avert my gaze as we trundled around the wards together.

In quite a short time Dr. Dinesh Rao in the absence of Georgina had become indispensable to the firm and I was growing in admiration of his qualities. It therefore came as quite a surprise when he asked me suddenly for a week's leave at extremely short notice.

'It may be difficult to cope with two of my junior staff away but I'll ask Mr. Mee, my consultant urology colleague, if we can share his houseman as I know his firm will be quiet next week as, I believe, he will be away himself.'

'I am sorry to have to ask for this without much warning but something has come up which is quite important for me.'

'Dr. Rao, I am sure you would not be asking me unless there was a very good reason so off you go and have a great time wherever it may be.'

To my slight irritation, Dr. Rao did not volunteer any more information as to where exactly he was planning to travel. No matter. I supposed I would hear about it all in due course.

The week he was absent went smoothly enough with the help and cooperation of the urology junior staff. The registrar kept a close eye on the problem patients which thankfully were few in number. Towards the end of the week a rumour began circulating that one of the other house surgeons had received a telephone call from Dinesh just before he was boarding a plane at Hong Kong airport. It appeared that he might be en route to somewhere else. What a dynamic fellow going all the way out to the Far East on only a week's leave! Jealously I wondered if the NHS were paying their senior house officers too generously.

Ten days later on Monday morning on the eight o'clock ward round I was relieved to see the whole team reassembled back safely from their travels.

'Thank Goodness you are all here at last. We have a hell of a week's work ahead of us,' I said teasing the youngsters on taking their well-deserved break.

'I am not envious, of course, but I hope you are both rested and had a great time.'

'Yes, we did actually!' replied Dinesh and Georgina almost in unison. This chorus in the affirmative took me a little by surprise but

I thought no more about it as we ploughed through the tasks of the morning. I had not noticed the slightly nervous laugh from Georgina that followed this joint statement. It was later I learnt of its significance. One thing I did observe was the fact that Dinesh's nasal boil had been substantially improved by the obvious exposure to sunlight in the eastern hemisphere. It no longer caught the eye and he was sporting a rather fine tan.

When the full story of that week emerged through leaked scraps of information it was a story of heroic proportion. Dr. Rao had risked everything on a whim. After he had asked for permission to take urgent leave, he had booked a flight to Sydney via Hong Kong and twenty-nine hours later was standing outside the outback ranch in New South Wales where Georgina was staying with her uncle. She had nearly collided with him as she had ridden back to the farmstead at full gallop after a day rounding up the cattle. To say she was startled might be an understatement. But she was not disappointed. After a few niceties Dinesh lost no time in showing her the reservation he had made for them both for a four day stay on Lady Elliot Island on the Great Barrier Reef.

After obtaining her uncle's agreement to be absent from the farm they drove back to Sydney and flew up to Brisbane and onto Bundaberg. From there a six-seater light aircraft took them the fifty miles to the hundred-acre coral cay that is Lady Elliot Island. It was on the plane that Dinesh made his first substantive move. He gently picked up Georgina's hand and laid it on his open palm.

'I hope you did not think me too forward but I have had this vision of taking you to a desert island for a long time. Lady Elliot is the nearest I could find. I hope you will think it as wonderful as I do being with you.'

Georgina smiled and made no effort to withdraw her hand. She stared not at the boil on his nose but into his large, kind, earnest brown eyes.

'Dinesh, this is the most romantic thing that has ever happened to me. How could I think it was anything but wonderful?'

Through the windows of the Piper aircraft came the vista that had been in Dinesh's mind these several months. A half mile wide coral island covered in plush vegetation surrounded by the whitest beach imaginable. A few wooden huts discreetly camouflaged in amongst the coconut trees near the larger of the island's two lagoons. In the afternoon sunshine it was the most beautiful thing that Georgina she had ever seen.

Certainly, enough to win any girl's heart.

Every day they had swum in the clear warm seas around the island. They had snorkelled close to reef sharks and spotted the gliding movement of a huge manta ray. They had been enthralled by the sight of green turtles crawling up the beach, digging their pits and laying their eggs in the moonlight. They had been startled by the screeching of the mutton birds from their sandy hollows near the cabin they were sleeping in. It had been the most magical time of their lives and much to remember when four days later they made the long journey back to the UK.

Months later, Dinesh and Georgina rotated out of my service to pursue their own paths in the maze that constitutes a medical career. I was sad to see them go but they were, in turn, replaced by competent successors.

Two years later they married and by the end of the decade a couple of children joined them. Dinesh went on to a career as a consultant plastic surgeon while Georgina with all her cheerfulness and charm became a GP and built a highly successful practice.

And it all started on my watch while we all cared together for 'the man who nearly died of pancreatitis.' Maybe there is something to be said for patronage and team spirit after all?

Back at Northwick Park life continued apace and time moved on. It seemed I was definitely part of the furniture as my practice began to grow. As a consultant I was still learning new ways of caring for my patients and soon I was given the chance soon to demonstrate this fact to a certain royal personage.

Chapter 9:
A Twenty-First Birthday Party

❖

As time passed at Northwick Park Hospital, I fell into the routines which would shape my practice for the next three decades. I learnt that there was no time to waste if all the tasks were to be accomplished. The ward rounds, the operating lists, the outpatient clinics and the vast amount of paperwork: All had to receive their due attention.

In addition, as with Georgina and Dinesh, there were the young doctors to train, students to teach, research projects to pursue and the need to cope with the large number of emergencies that a big hospital attracts. I discovered that setting my weekly programme to cope with all these demands was important and it was clear I must take a long view if I ever wanted to make an alteration to my schedule. In that sense it was much like driving an oil tanker. It takes a long time to set it going through the water and an awfully long time to stop or change course.

For example, if I wished to switch the timing of a particular weekly session it might take six months to engineer that change. It was vital to consider carefully if these changes were essential. My colleagues would indulge me to make a few changes to my programme but they would almost certainly not help me to change them back again if I found the new arrangements unsatisfactory.

Why is it so difficult to change a simple routine? The reason is that a surgeon's work is dependent on so many others. This is best illustrated by looking at the operating theatre where the list of essential people includes surgeon, anaesthetist, scrub nurse, assistant surgeon, operating department assistant, runner recovery nurse and porter, to name just a few. Even taking out an inflamed appendix requires at least a half-dozen trained workers.

To confuse it further, the chain of command has become blurred by government's insistence that it is all about team working. All very well and good but there has to be someone in charge to demand that the task is carried out in the first place. To initiate an operation, it has to be clear that the patient will suffer if the work is not done. It is not team work that decides who needs an operation but the surgeon sometimes with the help of a physician.

In this new post-deference world, it is precisely the failure of our non-expert political and administrative masters to understand this simple concept that has undermined the ability of the NHS to deliver. I am sure this applies as well to many other professions and businesses.

Administrators seem to be trained to undermine leadership roles at all times. Whether this is due to jealousy, malice or attending too many misguided management seminars I am not sure. The result is that working in socialised medicine, as the Americans term it, has become like swimming in treacle with no one person having the sense to pull the plug and go back to applying some of the good old-fashioned values that brought Western medicine to prominence in the first place.

But it is important not to look back with rose-tinted spectacles. Before the advent of the NHS in July 1948 there was great disparity and inequality in how resources and access to medical treatments were meted out. Access certainly improved after the NHS was born but it seems things have slipped a bit in recent years. We must be careful not to display 'first elevenitis', which is the common human foolishness that believes that all was bigger and better when we were young. It was not better in the good old days. Just different. When I was a houseman in the mid-seventies, I remember the waiting time for a hernia repair in my hospital on the NHS was four years. Ancillary workers were on strike as were some junior doctors and even the consultants joined in a go-slow to resist the then Labour government's Secretary of State for Health, Barbara Castle, who wanted to abolish private practice entirely from the NHS.

Despite trying hard, the NHS seems stuck with waiting lists, waiting times and inaccessibility. To change it seems impossible. Certainly, the so-called reforms of a generation ago have made only superficial improvements. More importantly it has disturbed the essential relationships in medicine between patients, doctors and nurses. Instead, we are all asked to look up to the politicians and their proxies who insist that they are responsible for the delivery of healthcare. A subject they do not, and cannot, know much about.

In those early years at Northwick Park Hospital, I did not think much on these difficulties. My job was to set up the structures that would support my service, attract and retain a loyal team of helpers and simply get on with it. It was absorbing work and I was single minded and focused on getting it right.

This task was temporarily interrupted by an important royal visitor.

***

Northwick Park Hospital was to celebrate its twenty-first birthday. It had been decided that, as Her Majesty the Queen had placed the foundation stone of the institution, one of her children, in this case Princess Anne, should be asked to witness its coming of age. She was to conduct a ward round and take a cup of tea with the staff. There was much debate as to how the Royal personage should spend the forty-five minutes she would be present in the hospital. Michael Cole, the Chief Executive, had got onto the case as soon as it had been agreed. He had set up a Royal Visit subcommittee to decide upon the details. I am sure they must have convened many important meetings to work it all out.

The Chairman of the Regional and the Area Health Authorities that had an interest, as well as the two local MPs, would join him to greet Her Royal Highness when she arrived. It was decided that the Chairman of the Medical Staff Committee and the Nursing Director should also be part of this entourage. After tea and a royal biscuit, the whole group would tour the wards and the outpatient department. The princess would pay a visit to the new Day Care Unit, after which the Her Highness would say a few choice words in the main lecture theatre to an invited audience. She would then present some long service medals before leaving.

It all seemed quite innocuous but led to much disruption for a week beforehand. Outpatient clinics were re-scheduled, elective admissions reduced, and metaphorical red carpets hired for the day. As for my role in all this excitement? I had been detailed to present a patient to the princess. We had just commenced keyhole surgery at the hospital so I was keen to show her the tiny incisions of one of my recovering gall-bladder patients. This lady had undergone a laparoscopic cholecystectomy where both the stones and her gall-bladder had been removed through four small incisions to prevent further attacks of biliary colic, the pain when the gall-bladder contracts half an hour after eating a meal.

It is satisfying surgery with good results and the laparoscopic operation has quickly become the routine approach for this condition. Its advantage is that the patient has minimal scarring from the four stab incisions so the patient enjoys a much quicker recovery. In those days in the early 1990s when the procedure, pioneered in France and introduced via the USA, was being adopted by British surgeons, learning the procedure from scratch was arduous. Consultant surgeons often operated together for moral support to familiarize themselves with the new skills required. With the image of the patient's gall-bladder displayed on a TV screen it was often the case of looking at the monitor and deciding together the next move.

There were plenty of frustrations with the equipment as the image often failed or the laparoscope got misted up. We would also find that the gall-bladders would not always oblige us by displaying normal anatomy. In consequence we would have to convert to the old open method with a six-inch incision with all the morbidity that follows. Occasionally the laparoscopic method would take three or four hours of fiddling about before the gall-bladder could be removed safely. In recent years this operating time has been reduced significantly and today it rarely takes more than an hour.

I was due to remove Mrs. Green's gall-bladder on the Thursday and the princess was to visit the next day. I had briefed the patient who had agreed to shake the royal hand and I had laid out a set of the new instruments for HRH to inspect. It would be a pleasant change from my usual routine and I was looking forward to it. I had donned a fresh white coat (it was another eighteen years before white coats for medical staff were to be mysteriously banned by the Department of Health). I made sure that I wore my identification badge and I even got Christina to cut my hair.

When Thursday came, I was a little nervous about Mrs. Green's gall-bladder operation. It was all so new. The first laparoscopic cholecystectomies in the UK had been performed at St. Mary's Hospital in Paddington in late 1991. In front of an audience of hundreds of surgeons the operations had not gone perfectly. One of the cases had resulted in disaster. The surgeons watching had all witnessed an eminent surgeon damage a common bile duct causing serious injury to the patient.

The operation on Mrs. Green was my twelfth operation of this type. I knew all about gall-bladder surgery as I had previously taken out three hundred of them by the open, large incision, method. But the laparoscopic approach was awkward as we were operating eighteen inches away from the surgical field with few ways to control bleeding. Someone described it once as chopstick surgery. The lack of touch, or haptic perception as it is termed, was frightening for a relative novice.

I was pleased to have my senior registrar operating with me that day. A man of my own age who like me had struggled to progress in his career, he was waiting to take up his consultant post in East Anglia. He had taken on the new surgery eagerly and was trying to become proficient. We were both aware of the dangers of new methods in unskilled hands and we both feared the bizarre complications that had been described elsewhere.

But in Mrs. Green's case the operation had all gone to plan and I was confident that she would go home the next day after meeting the princess.

***

My own prior experience with the laparoscope had been more than a dozen years before. It might therefore be assumed I must be an expert by the time of the royal visit but that first experience was a catastrophe.

I was working as a young surgical registrar in Basingstoke and one weekend I admitted a young woman with suspected appendicitis. For most of my professional life I have been hunting out inflamed appendixes. Despite it being a common illness, making the diagnosis is not straightforward. Over the years I have tried, like all my colleagues to avoid missing seriously inflamed appendixes while, at the same time, not taking out normal ones unnecessarily. Even today we have no reliable test to define whether an appendix is inflamed. Ultrasound examination and CT scan have been only partially effective with many false negatives reducing the overall diagnostic accuracy. I had heard of this new instrument, the laparoscope, which afforded a quick look to see if the appendix was inflamed. If it was then out it would come with three small incisions. If not, it would stay where it belonged.

That weekend on call in Hampshire in 1978 I had a patient who was an ideal guinea pig for this new advance. She was very tender on the right side and had some signs of toxaemia. However, the history was not quite right. It was entirely possible that she might have mittelschmerz (mid-cycle pain) or salpingitis (inflamed tubes) both of which are best treated expectantly or with antibiotics.

I had learnt that there was a gynaecology registrar in the hospital and that she was a whizz with this new laparoscopic method. The technique had been pioneered by Karl Semm, a gynaecologist himself, in Germany and was allowing colleagues to make much more accurate diagnoses. I bleeped her and told her of my case and asked if she might assist to show me the new technique. I had the impertinence to ask her how many she had carried out before. She said she had performed nearly three hundred. I was therefore confident it would be safe. She reassured me further when she said she was submitting a paper on the technique to the British Medical Journal.

A couple of hours later our patient was consented and asleep on the operating table. A relaxing anaesthetic meant that the abdominal wall muscles were floppy and would give us good access to the peritoneal cavity inside. To begin laparoscopy a needle is inserted through a small incision below the umbilicus and carbon dioxide under pressure insufflated into the abdominal cavity. The abdomen distends so that a full and safe view of the organs within is revealed.

We painted and draped the patient and my gynaecological colleague made a small incision close to the belly button. She inserted a long Veress needle with a spring guarded point that protects the underlying intestines after passing through the muscle and fascia of the abdominal wall. Once into the cavity a pressure drop or fall of resistance demonstrates that one is inside the peritoneal cavity. Then three or four litres of carbon dioxide are pumped in to maintain pressure. This was achieved without difficulty and the registrar then picked up a large sharp, rather terrifying looking trocar and plunged it into the ballooned, distended abdomen.

It was all so effortless and, as it was my case, I determined to be the first one to look in and see whether the appendix was ripe for removal. I placed my right eye to the eyepiece attached to the end of the eighteen-inch laparoscopic fibre-optic lens and looked within.

I could see nothing but red.

'Needs a bit of washing at the end, I think. Is it always so red? You have a look,' I said.

She looked in and I saw her confidence sap from her. She went as white as a sheet. Just at that moment the anaesthetist added loudly from the top end of the table that the patient's blood pressure had dropped.

'Er, I think I may have gone into a major vessel!' the gynaecological registrar moaned.

'Hell, I think we have a major bleeding problem here. We've got to open her pronto!' I yelled.

I called for a scalpel and incised quickly in the midline. At the same time, I shouted to the scrub nurse.

'Please call my consultant Mr. Heald at home for me and ask him to come to theatre immediately if he would!'

No longer in command of the operation the poor gynaecology registrar was assisting me, the general surgical registrar, who really did not have enough skill to cope with the unfolding problem. Within two minutes I had the contents of the abdomen displayed and I sucked out nearly a litre of dark blood. There was a hole in the front of the right common iliac vein as it entered the pelvis. Blood was welling up rapidly like some slow bubbling geyser.

It was going to be right at the edge of my competence to be able to stop this bleeding and save this young woman's life.

'5/0 vascular prolene sutures and some venous clamps please as quick as you can, sister!'

'I think I have some digital pressure control now! Sucker sister! Get some O negative blood up to theatre immediately and cross-match six more units please!' I shouted to my anaesthetist.

I was pretty scared.

'Pelvic packs please! Now let's have the side clamps and the prolene sutures!'

'OK! Side clamp on and I am suturing the vessel!'

Within five more minutes I had a continuous proline suture repair of the vein completed and I released the clamp. It stayed dry. Job done! I had been lucky that my youthful, clumsy surgical manoeuvres had not torn the wall of the vein further.

'Right let's look at the appendix!'

I pulled up the caecum and behind it was a very nasty, thickened and quite smelly appendix with a small perforation leaking pus and a little stool.

'Well, at least we have the right diagnosis at last. Let's take it out!'

As we did so my consultant strode in to theatre a little out of breath.

'Do you have control Peter? Good. I'll just scrub up and check for you as I know you have not done much vascular surgery. OK?'

'Thank you very much, Mr. Heald.'

Five minutes later the repair in the vessel had been checked and the filthy appendix was in the bucket. For the first time in twenty-five minutes, we could relax. We calmed down by chatting about what had happened. Ten minutes later the consultant had left for home and I was closing the wound.

It had not been a happy hour and a half.

As I look back at my first experience of laparoscopy twelve years before the laparoscopic revolution began to change the face of abdominal surgery, I am not surprised that I was not an early adopter of the new technology. The method that led to the crisis that day of the Veress needle technique and the blind trocar placement is still in use today but I have always been distrustful of this 'closed' method. I use an 'open' method where I make a small incision and place a blunt trocar gently into the peritoneal cavity. Not very elegant sometimes, but a deal safer.

I hope that gynaecology registrar changed her method of inserting the laparoscope to the open method after that fateful night in 1978.

***

It was the open method I had used on Mrs. Green the day before Princess Anne was due to meet her. After entry to the peritoneum was achieved safely the carbon dioxide distended the abdomen. I then dissected out the gall-bladder with a hook and a diathermy current passing down it to cut the tissues and coagulate the vessels when they bled.

Carefully I defined the cystic duct, the narrow tube that connects the gall-bladder to the common bile duct. I double clipped both it and the artery with four small titanium clips and removed the gall-bladder from its bed under the liver. I kept in the right plane to avoid unnecessary bleeding from the liver and to avoid a leak of bile from an accessory biliary duct. Finally I popped the now free-floating gallbladder into a plastic bag and pulled it out through the incision near the belly button. On this occasion there was little bleeding and no technical difficulties.

The whole procedure took just over an hour.

On the morning of the princess' ward round Mrs. Green was a bit sore but had already polished off a hearty breakfast when I checked up on her.

'Good, Mrs. Green, I am glad to see you are looking well. Still keen to meet the princess?'

'Very happy Mr. McDonald and then home later if possible?' she added.

'Yes, of course.'

At exactly 4.30pm, I was standing at the entrance to Mrs. Green's cubicle feeling almost as nervous as I did in that operating theatre back in 1978. The entourage was heading around the corner of the ward preceded by a photographer from The Harrow Observer. There were several people I had never seen before but Michael Cole accompanying Princess Anne put me at my ease.

'Your Royal Highness I would like you to meet Mr. McDonald, one of our newer consultants, who would like to show you a patient from whom he removed a gall-bladder yesterday by the new keyhole method, ma'am.'

A royal hand was gently stretched out towards me and I shook it gently. I pondered just how many it had shaken in its lifetime.

'Please come this way Your Royal Highness and meet Mrs. Green. She is recovering well after her operation yesterday morning. It took just sixty-five minutes and was a success. Her gall-bladder and its stones had caused her a great deal of pain in recent months. Here they are in a jar and laid out on the trolley are some of the instruments used in the operation.'

Her Royal Highness winced considerably while I was explaining the procedure. She peered with distaste as she eyed up the jar with the gall-bladder floating like some ghostly jelly fish in amongst the stones.

'All done through very tiny incisions. I can show you them, ma'am. I am sure you would be interested to see them?'

I was just about to pull back the sheets and display Mrs. Green's tummy when Princess Anne quickly intervened.

'No, no, no! Mr. McDonald that will not be necessary!'

'Of course, ma'am!'

'Well done Mrs. Green,' continued the royal personage, 'when are you going home?'

'When you have finished with me Your Royal Highness!'

'Well, that will be very shortly. Well done to you and Mr. McDonald and his team. Goodbye and thank-you.'

With that the photographer' camera flashed and the party moved on to the next ward. Michael Cole winked and smiled at me as he walked past. The group started to move off down to the other end of the ward.

The twenty-first birthday visit was over and within another half hour the hospital returned to normal. Mrs. Green got home courtesy of her husband to a future without biliary colic. Later I sent her a framed photograph of her and Princess Anne to hang in her sitting room. On the wall of my office at Northwick Park Hospital is a print of Princess Anne standing next to me at the end of Mrs. Green's bed. I have used it in many lectures to joke that doctors who train with me come from all walks of life. This bad joke is greeted with a polite chuckle and sighs of disbelief.

But, at least, it allows me to recall that twenty-first birthday party in 1991 when my afternoon routine was enlivened by a royal visit. It was nice to have been part of an old tradition where royals open buildings and applaud good works.

Britain at its best, some might say, but I never lost sight of the fact that I was working now in one of the most cosmopolitan part of the British Isles. With a third of my patients having been born outside the UK, I was always aware that tradition for them meant something often quite different.

Chapter 10:
The Melting Pot

❖

The hospital at Northwick Park in Harrow looks after as diverse a population as anywhere in Britain. The history of London over the last two millennia has been a history of migration and of immigration.

From the countryside and from abroad and then out again to the shires.

Although many different nationalities were to be found in medieval London, it was not until the middle of the nineteenth century that large numbers of strangers from strange lands came pouring in. Scots, Irish, Jews, Francophones, Spaniards, Latin Americans, Portuguese and Brazilians, West Indians, Africans, Pakistanis, Indians, Sri Lankans, Greeks, Cypriots, Turks, Italians, Chinese, and more recently Somalis, Bosnians, Syrians, Afghanis and Russians.

Generally speaking, there have been relatively few problems between these groups. Britain has experienced race riots rarely and it can be said that integration of these new groups has been steady. London has ghettos but there is enough contact between groups to stop misunderstandings getting out of hand. Certainly, we have never experienced the extremes of ethnic friction seen by our continental colleagues in the past century.

At the level of the hospital these new immigrants bring a few problems. Not only do we see new patterns of disease but an army of interpreters is required to help communicate with the newcomers. These polyglots are needed almost any time of the day or night. Occasionally we are forced to get one on the phone instead of in person. An imperfect solution in most doctors' opinion and one I have yet to try myself.

I learnt quite quickly that a ward round at Northwick Park was often an interesting affair as there would always be half a dozen patients with no English at all. I saw this as a challenge rather than an irritant as I have always enjoyed speaking lots of languages very badly.

'Namaste!' would always go down well with the Gujuratis who had come from East Africa. Their now grown-up children speak English perfectly but some of the older generation still have not mastered it after forty years.

'Dukhavo?'

'Thodu, thodu! Bahu saru!'

'Avjo!'

However inappropriate my attempts were, these faltering words always broke the ice and a large smile would appear on the face of the patient. I looked the part too as I have what my wife calls 'full features'. Years ago, when I was travelling overland in Asia I was often mistaken for an Afghan or a Turk. I have a swarthy skin inherited from a maternal great-great grandfather who was said to have come over to England from Tunisia. He was clearly a freeloader as he left my great grandmother with two children and little money to live in Birmingham before he beetled back to North Africa.

Starting with a Hindu greeting but receiving no response, 'salam alekum!' would closely follow just in case I had misjudged on which side of the religious divide the patient belonged. If they were Muslim a bright 'alekum salam!' would be communicated in return.

A year spent wandering at twenty across Asia to India has not been wasted as it has given me an insight into the lives of many of the patients I now treat. Many run small businesses all around Northwest London with varying degrees of success. Asian accountants, Jewish financiers, Greek barbers, Bangladeshi restauranteurs, Iranian traders and first generation British/Gujurati computer programmers.

As I look around the mix of races where I work, I think of my paternal great grandfather, George Bruce McDonald. Another immigrant and the only other doctor in the family. He had qualified in Glasgow in 1864. I still possess his diploma in medicine signed by his professor of surgery, one Joseph Lister. George had migrated south to London and was employed close to where I now work. He practised as a mental health physician at St. Bernard's Hospital Asylum in Hanwell. Once called the Middlesex Asylum, its remains are next door to the modern hospital at Ealing where I sometimes operate.

The Middlesex Asylum was a pioneering establishment deciding to discard straight-jackets and restraints for controlling unruly patients. The doctors and nurses substituted kindness and common-sense when treating the insane. By doing so they pioneered the modern approach to psychiatric illness.

When I drive into the car park at Ealing, I observe all the different races who make up the patients and staff of the modern hospital. I reflect how the people would have looked for my great-grandfather when he began his work there in his black tail coat and beard. A world away from my current Harris Tweed jacket and sometimes tieless shirt.

Although I make a lot of effort to speak in rough French, Italian, Spanish, German, Gujurati and Hindi I find myself emulating a previous consultant I worked for. Bob Lane was a fine surgeon but an eccentric character who, it was rumoured, had been to acting school before studying medicine. Certainly, his sense of theatre was well developed and not just theatre of the surgical kind. When performing an operation to replace a leaking abdominal aorta with a graft, he would release the vascular clamp from this great vessel with a grand gesture to test its patency. As he did so he would shout at the top of his voice in the manner of Long John Silver.

'Ooooh Aaaagh! Mind your eyes!'

He would accompany this exhortation by singing two verses of Rule Britannia as the spurt of blood would hit the theatre light two foot above our heads demonstrating just how well he had unblocked the artery ready to sew in the graft to the downstream aorta.

But this much admired and singular surgeon made one major discovery that I still employ today. It is the fact that, if you talk to patients in their own accents, it improves their comprehension when their knowledge of English is poor. At first sight this might seem disrespectful, even denigrating, but in my experience, it is highly successful and its motive is never misinterpreted. Moreover, the patients seem to love the improvement in communication it affords.

I learnt recently that this is called 'code-switching' and we all do this to a greater or lesser extent when we talk to others. Even in our own mother tongues. When we are in a group with a common but strong regional English accent, we tend to talk more like the group. Indeed, we unconsciously mimic each other to conform. The converse is that when we encounter a group with so-called received English/accentless pronunciation, we all talk more precisely and avoid vernacular slang.

It is simply a case of trying to improve our chances of being understood.

And communication is everything in medicine.

Back to my theatrical boss.

When an Austrian frau who had never quite mastered English presented with abdominal pain to his outpatient clinic, he would ask in a thick Teutonic accent:

'Und wo ist der painz, mein Frau Schmidt?'

The patients' face would light up as she replied while vigorously pointing to her tummy.

'Und hier, und hier und hier, Herr Arzt!'

It would be the same with a Chinese waiter.

In a breathless Cantonese accent he would enquire.

'Oo, Aa, Ha, Ho war is dare pain? Ha, why?'

Even old farmers from the depths of the Hampshire countryside near where he worked were not exempt if he considered that a question in a colloquial accent would be helpful. He would blurt out to them with a wry smile.

'Oooh Aaaaah! Oooh Aaaaah! Noice to see yar, Farmarr Smith! Doo yoo have any pains?'

Funny though it seems his method always worked. Indeed, there is some scientific data to show that this method, now called the chameleon effect, puts the other person at their ease. Someone once demonstrated scientifically that a Frenchman will understand an

English speaker better if a Gallic accent is used. So, it is reasonable to use lots of 'veez' and 'errrrs' and pouting of the lips as you speak in English to a Frenchman while waving your arms around.

Not only in the melting pot of Northwick Park was there the language to consider but the cultural and behavioural differences between the groups was real and could not be ignored. Political correctness suggests we should pretend these differences are minimal or even non-existent. That is surely ridiculous. Allowance must be given for these variations in national personality.

As a medical student I remember being struck by how different the background noise was in the labour wards of the obstetric unit in Bedford Hospital compared with the noisy ones in Venezuela where I did a three month student elective. Although the ease of delivery for 'las donnas' in Venezuela should be greater due their multiparous habits, most having at least four or five children, the act of delivery was staggeringly distinct.

In Bedford the ladies gritted their teeth, squeezed their husbands' fingers to the point of fracture, whimpered a little while sobbing with pleasure at the final denouement. Often they would apologise if they had made a little noise as if it was forbidden.

By contrast in Venezuela, where I delivered babies in the little coastal town of Guiria, within sight of the island of Trinidad, the volume and length of their screams were blood curdling. Their gritas would reach a crescendo and be amplified by the corrugated iron roof of the hospital. Only a thunderstorm and its deafening patter of rain could drown out their screeches. It was a dramatic and noisy affair.

Each race has a different story to tell and there is a great deal of difference as to how they express the physical or mental changes that disease may demand from them.

***

This was certainly the case for Mrs. Andra Patel. Like many of her friends she was overweight at fifty. As an aficionado of Indian cuisine, I have always sympathised with this. Indian food is so delicious and nutritious but also very fattening. I have spent a lot of time in my clinics urging my Asian patients to lose weight before their complex operations as they do better post-operatively when they start as slimmer models.

'Cut out the chapatis!' I urge them.

'But I eat very little, doctor!' they chorus back.

Although Andra had tried hard to put similar advice into practice, the lure of rice and roti always seemed to beat her. She had never really succeeded to lose weight despite years of restraint. That was until the year before I saw her. The weight loss started with an attack of gastroenteritis when visiting her mother and father back in India. However, it never really settled. The diarrhoea continued and, by the time she went to see her doctor about her worries, she was ten kilograms lighter than before.

Dr. Lloyd was the doyen of our local GPs in Northwest London. A man with the energy of five of his colleagues, he was the local GP trainer as well as having set up an on-call service of colleagues when the government allowed GP practices to opt-out from covering the emergencies.

When Andra was brought into his consulting room by her husband that morning he knew immediately she needed admission to hospital.

'Hello, Mrs. Patel. Now you don't look too well to me. How long has this been going on?'

'Dr. Lloyd, I have had this diarrhoea for months now and it is getting worse and worse. Now there is blood in the stool as well. And I have to rush like mad to visit the toilet.'

'How often do you have to go?' asked the good doctor.

'Maybe twenty times a day and five times at night! Now I am so weak I can hardly get out of bed without the help of my husband.'

'I see. Let's have a look at you.'

David examined Mrs. Patel thoroughly and did not like what he saw. The middle-aged woman was clearly wasting away. Dehydrated, anaemic, cachectic, weak. Her pulse was fast and her breathing pretty rapid.

'I do not like the look of you at all, Mrs. Patel so I am going to get you into the hospital today.'

'Really? But I have my daughter's wedding in six weeks' time. I cannot be ill at this time!'

'We'll have to see if they can get you back to health before that. But you cannot go on like this.'

A few phone calls and four hours later Mrs. Patel was in the medical ward at Northwick Park Hospital. Blood had been sent to the laboratory and had shown that her haemoglobin and albumin levels were extremely low. A drip had been set up and blood was ordered. A doctor had felt her tummy and looked up her bottom. An X-ray had followed and some stool sent off to the lab for culture.'

A gastroenterology opinion was sought. A diagnosis of ulcerative colitis was made and intravenous steroids started at high dose. Mrs. Patel still felt completely rotten though she considered she was now in safe hands.

The next day I got a phone call from the gastroenterologist.

'Hi Peter, Meron here. I would like your help with a patient. A Mrs. Patel on Gaskell Ward. Fulminant ulcerative colitis with a toxic megacolon. No growth from stools. Blood transfusion, high dose IV hydrocortisone and we just started that new medicine infliximab as there is some evidence that it works in this circumstance. But she still might need surgery soon so come and give me your opinion.'

What Meron, the gastroenterologist, was requesting I had heard a dozen times before. No-one knows what causes ulcerative colitis and why one patient gets it more severely than another. The lining of the colon falls away leaving its interior surface resembling a severe burn. In consequence the colon leaks large quantities of blood and protein and, because it can no longer absorb fluid, copious diarrhoea, low protein levels and anaemia follow. Eventually if the disease process worsens the colon blows up like a balloon and the patient may die of severe dehydration, or the colon may perforate leading to peritonitis and death.

The object of surgical intervention is to pre-empt those last stages. Only 10% of patients with ulcerative colitis ever need an operation as most attacks can be managed with a variety of medical treatments. Corticosteroids, such as hydrocortisone, have been the main drugs used over the last fifty years but in recent years immunosuppressives and monoclonal antibodies, the miracle drugs used in tumours and chronic inflammations, have been successfully employed.

Repairing the damage to the colon is therefore a priority as it avoids an operation. With Mrs. Patel it was a case of treating hard and fast while waiting for improvement.

But Mrs. Patel's colon did not respond to the drugs. This was the reason Meron had called me to get me involved. My task was neither to operate unnecessarily nor operate too late. A tall order. But if a gastroenterologist of his experience was asking me to see her there was a damn good chance an operation was what she would eventually need.

After introducing myself that afternoon, I saw her again the next morning on my ward round. There were couple of nurses helping so I was able to get much more information second-hand as they busied around her. Nothing they said reassured me. There had been no improvement overnight at all. My impression now was that this was a woman who needed an operation very soon.

Despite being ill Mrs. Patel was able to give me polite responses to my questions. This cheered me because, although she was septic and malnourished, it seemed to me that she would have enough strength to get through the operation.

I looked at the parameters that we judge the severity of an attack of ulcerative colitis. Pulse, temperature, anaemia, blood in the stools, raised inflammatory markers, stool frequency and abdominal pain are all taken into account.

For Mrs. Patel it was time to take the big step.

'Would you like me to talk to your husband with you?' I asked.

'Please. He's in the corridor outside the ward,' she replied weakly.

With her husband present, I began to explain where we were. Mrs. Patel's parlous physical state was due to her illness. Sepsis, lack of protein, muscle wasting and a low blood pressure. All signs of impending gram-negative septicaemia. As I explained this I wondered if she had already suffered a small perforation of her colon, partly walled off in the peritoneum by the surrounding organs.

I was sure now that her colon needed to come out as it was just not responding to the medicines and the general support.

That was the bad news.

The good news was that ever since Sir William Allchin in 1885 described the first fatal case of acute fulminating ulcerative colitis, it has been known that only the colon is involved in this condition and that other organs are spared. This distinguishes it from its sister condition of Crohn's disease. So, Mrs. Patel would undoubtedly be cured by the operation, or operations, I was proposing.

I explained that to save her life I must remove her colon, leaving the rectum in place, and fashion an ileostomy, an opening of the small bowel onto the abdomen. This would be the first stage and then when she was back to full health again in six months, we could discuss the further options.

The Patels looked crestfallen but they were brave souls and I guessed they would cope well. In some groups, such as Middle Eastern Arabs and some Africans, the idea of being left with an ileostomy and a bag on the surface of the abdomen, a stoma as it is called, is seen as a worse fate than dying. This makes the decision to operate to save life that much harder.

I was relieved to note the Patels were not in this group so I continued with my reassurance.

'You will quickly get used to the stoma and you will not find it too much of a burden. You will, of course, be in good health again after months of feeling awful.'

They did not seem very impressed by my explanation but I continued.

'We can operate this evening if you give your consent and you will be feeling a million times better by the morning.'

I was not lying.

Out of all the operations I have performed in my surgical career, emergency total colectomy and ileostomy for colitis is my favourite. The reason is that within a few hours it changes a dying patient to a living, recovering one. A miracle performed by mere mortals.

'OK Mr. McDonald, please go ahead with the operation as soon as you can,' the Patels sighed together.

With the decision made we carried on with our ward round while the nurses and doctors prepared Mrs. Patel for her operation.

***

It began at five-thirty and it took two hours. An incision was made in the midline and the intestines exposed. The colon was grossly distended, flaccid and dull looking but thankfully there was no perforation. This reassured me that Mrs. Patel's post-operative recovery would be rapid and hopefully uneventful.

I divided the mesentery of the colon bit-by-bit between Spencer-Wells clamps allowing the registrar on-call for the night to tie his surgical knots carefully to seal the not insubstantial blood vessels that feed the colon. With that done I ran a linear-cutter across the terminal ileum and the sigmoid colon, just upstream to the rectum, and passed the now-separated colon to the scrub nurse to send to the pathologists for later analysis.

A trephine, a hole, was made in the right iliac fossa of the abdomen, the appendix area, and the divided 'active' end of the ileum brought out. The abdomen was closed in layers and the ileostomy was fashioned into a spout. This spout, which appears to worsen the cosmetic aspect of having a stoma, was to make sure the small bowel content, which contains many corrosive enzymes, had minimal contact with the skin. In this way it avoids excoriation, soreness or even ulceration of the skin around the stoma.

The operation was over and the patient headed for a night in surgical high-care before she went back to the ward the next day.

Over the next six days Mrs. Patel's progress was rapid. Within three days she was beginning to eat and drink and all her intravenous lines were removed. The strong medicines that had failed to control the inflammation in the colon were tailed off. She was mobilising well and was beginning to gain weight for the first time in months. Her wound was clean and healing and when I saw her next, she was asking when she might go home.

'Soon, I think. Soon,' I reassured.

Five days after her surgery I was reviewing her again.

'Mr. McDonald did you now Mrs. Patel's daughter is getting married in four weeks' time? I know it might be difficult but will she be OK for that do you think?' asked a staff nurse.

'Yes, I did know and I think it will be fine, staff nurse,' I replied.

'But won't they all see my stoma?' moaned the patient.

'I am sure you will be able to wear your best sari and no-one needs to know about anything, Mrs. Patel. Obviously, you may have to ask others to do some of the running around as you will not be up to full strength for about three months. But I am sure they will understand. We will get my house surgeon to organise any occupational and stoma therapy and your GP will help you get what you need.'

When Mrs. Patel went home the next day her bed was quickly filled with another colitis sufferer from the same community. For unknown reasons, it has been noted that South Asians after they settle in the UK have a higher chance of developing ulcerative colitis. A mystery indeed and one that I hope will be solved one day.

I did not lose touch with Mrs. Patel. I monitored her monthly in outpatients. She told me how wonderful her daughter's wedding weekend had been but that she had wisely retired early to bed each night.

After three months she was really well and had put much of her weight back on but was keen to keep below the obesity threshold.

We began discussing her next options.

I explained that the rectum needed removing as it can be a site for a later cancer or more troublesome recurrent colitis. I could make a new rectum out of small intestine, an ileal pouch, and join it to the anus and later close her ileostomy. Two more operations certainly but it meant she would be able to dispense with the ileostomy and all its bags. Alternatively, I could remove the rectum and anus and leave her as she was. This is often the procedure of choice in the elderly as the second and third operations are not without their complications and risks.

Mrs. Patel opted for the ileal pouch and six months later I re-organised her plumbing and after a few more weeks with the ileostomy closed surgically in a third operation, she was passing motions through her anus.

When next I saw her, she gave me a huge grin and a pair of ornate Indian pyjamas. She knew I was familiar with her homeland and I had always found this style of evening wear very comfortable.

'Thank you, Mrs. Patel! What a great present!'

'No Mr. McDonald thank-you for giving me my life back!'

And so, ended another small chapter in my life at Northwick Park, but it was not the end of the pyjama story. On two more separate occasions over the next five years a parcel would arrive for me at the hospital from an Indian tailor in Wembley with yet another pair of kurta and pyjama.

It is for this reason alone that for many years Christina has noticed that I have dressed for bed like a Maharaja.

Chapter 11: Scribbling

❖

Life as a surgeon is often taxing but almost always rewarding. Everyone has their own method of coping with stress in a job. Some may moan in coffee rooms while others may go for a vigorous run after work. My catharsis has been scribbling. I have always written diaries and have published as many opinion pieces as I have been able. I have managed to turn this coping mechanism into a part-time career.

Although I have greatly enjoyed expressing myself it has often got me into trouble with the medical establishment.

My childhood had equipped me well to be a scribbler.

My father was a lover of words and spent his whole life reading when he was not working as a surveyor. He explained words and their derivations. He talked of ancient civilisations and their histories. His knowledge was encyclopaedic. He was an admired raconteur with a clever wit but as far as I remember he never wrote anything down much. I liked what I heard orally from him but vowed that, when my time came, I would not just read but write as well.

My mother gave me the other essential quality a writer must have: Never be frightened of argument or criticism. She was a contrarian who loved controversy. She gloried in being provocative and she was always keen to start a debate. In her own way she was fearless. She could talk to anyone. She could squabble with anyone. She was annoyingly great fun to be with. A good role model because a scribbler must be willing to provoke and by provoking accept any debate which follows. I have inherited that trait so much that my second son calls me 'The Great Polemicist'.

By scribbling I was following a well-trodden medical tradition. Many doctors have written successfully over the centuries and, although I do not claim to be in the same league, I must mention Conan Doyle, Chekhov, AJ Cronin, Erasmus, Darwin, Smollett, and even St. Luke, to name just seven.

My scribbling habit began as a medical student when I became a roving reporter for the student newspaper at University College Hospital. I was insanely inquisitive even as a young man. I remember interviewing and writing about a new organisation called GaySoc, which was one of the first student societies helping homosexuals come out into the open. It is extraordinary to reflect now on how ignorant we all were about such things in those days in the late sixties. My little piece made quite a stir.

Even more daring was an exclusive with Michael X, who was the British West Indian equivalent of Malcolm X in the United States. He was a rather frightening character and there was an undercurrent of violence in what he was saying to the young buck reporter who sat in front of him. Although I was certainly out of my comfort zone, I wrote something rather racy for the magazine. I was the intrepid investigative reporter telling it how it was. I gained some kudos from the piece but my subject, Michael X, came to a very sticky end just a few years later.

The financial life of most scribblers is precarious to say the least unless you are in that rare special league. Writers basically do not make money. It was said by a wit that a successful writer is one who earns over £10,000, in today's money, from their writing. I can confidently say I have never achieved that. Like one of my sons Archie, who is struggling to earn a living as a musician, writing is very competitive and terribly badly paid. Each year it seems to pay less. Fees for freelance articles in real terms have been drifting downwards year after year. Indeed, my highest paid freelance article of all time was published in 1978 and that figure of £385 for a 1,500-word magazine article is never likely to be bettered. In today's money that sum would now be £2,200. I must have felt like a king.

But like music, writing has an important secondary purpose. The cleansing of the mind and the soul. It is a means of processing the confusion around us and, in a small way, influencing the world in which we live. By doing so it has enabled me to understand more and cope better. I sometimes feel as a writer, I am like a satellite looking down on the surface of the planet sending pulses of critical energy to anywhere and to anyone I choose. And it makes me feel better.

My writing for the medical press is a form of self-criticism of my profession, hinting at change and reform.

Anton Chekhov, a general practitioner, and afterwards a world-famous playwright wrote:

'Doctors are the same as lawyers; the only difference is that lawyers merely rob you, whereas doctors rob you and kill you, too!'

A cynical view of our trade forcing us doctors, as well as the lawyers, to speculate on our true worth.

Writing, of course, can sometimes be criticism without responsibility and that is one of its weaknesses. Almost a cowardly act but one with a long pedigree. Pointing out flaws in systems is easy. It takes not much time or effort. Running the organisation that the scribbler is criticising, is much harder. Managing anything is always a hard, imperfect business. Writers must never forget that fact when they sharpen their critical pencils.

But there is yet another rationale to writing.

Voltaire (1694-1778), who was not a doctor, once wrote that: 'The purpose of Medicine is to amuse while nature takes its course.'

This has been one of my other aims in scribbling much as I have used humour to cheer my patients through their illnesses. The corollary of this is that by amusing both my readers and my patients I have cheered myself up at the same time.

I began to write for a variety of medical and other magazines often on medical subjects, or the politics and philosophies underpinning the medical world: *World Medicine*, *Pulse*, *She*, *The Times*, and *Geographical*. I learnt the hard lessons of frequent rejection as well as the exhilaration of having an article accepted and receiving those small cheques as pocket money. Finally, I landed a weekly column in a professional publication called Hospital Doctor. Despite its parochial constituency it had 40,000 regular readers to whom I could vent my spleen. This was a true catharsis as I tried to climb the career ladder in surgery.

I wrote of the flaws of the medical system and pointed out its inequality, unfairness and hypocrisy. I wrote about consultants who bullied and patients who abused the system. When the medical politicians erred I was ready to point out their foibles.

I had fun plagiarising greater writers:

'All the world's a stage
And all the doctors and surgeons merely players
They have their diagnoses and their therapies
And hospital doctors in their time play many parts
Their careers being in Seven Ages…' …etc.
(With apologies to William Shakespeare)

Occasionally my natural exuberance would backfire badly and the establishment would threaten to cut me down to size.

Once I reported on an open meeting in my hospital where a knighted Chairman of the Regional Health Authority was laying down his new policies. He had been invited by the senior surgeon to address all the consultants and trainees in Southampton where I worked. I wrote what I thought was an amusing and analytical piece highlighting his thinking and proposals. But in a moment of cheeky indiscretion, I described him as a man with the 'unmistakable accent of someone not brought up on a housing estate.'

I knew I might have stepped over the mark by writing that phrase but, as it amused me so much, I suspected it would amuse my readers too. It was not long before the senior consultant, who was a bombastic fellow, read it.

I had learnt previously that anything I scribbled, that was in any way critical of an individual, even though I never mentioned names, would be relayed back to them. Usually, it was their worst enemy in the hospital who would insist on showing it to them.

The senior consultant inwardly digested my article and went ballistic as he felt his personal integrity had been besmirched. He phoned me up and yelled: 'How dare you write about that meeting,

Mr. McDonald! It was a private meeting. Don't you think it is about time you decided whether you want to be a surgeon or a third-rate writer? You have embarrassed the whole hospital!'

It was a vicious telling off for me at a time when I needed the support of my seniors to progress. Although it was the first time, I had heard that a meeting outlining plans for the distribution and expenditure of public money was private, I took his point. I lost plenty of sleep that week as I mulled over what I should do to put things right. From time to time when my writing has hit its mark, it usually means it is relevant and correct. The reaction to it, in consequence, can be very harsh. I have tried to become thicker skinned over the years but it has not been easy.

That week was particularly difficult for me.

Not yet married to Christina I had no-one to lean on. After much soul-searching, I decided the only sensible course of action to diffuse the criticism was to telephone the chairman's office and apologise to him personally. This was a brave undertaking for an employee of the hospital, a doctor like me at the ordinary rank of registrar. To seek out and apologise to the Chairman of the Regional Board would be a terribly hard task but I had to do it.

With trepidation I picked up the telephone.

'Er, is that the Regional Chairman's Office?' I asked hesitatingly, hardly able to articulate the words.

'Yes, who may I ask is calling, sir?' came the reply.

'It's Dr. Peter McDonald from Southampton. I would be grateful if I could speak to the chairman personally. I need to apologise about an article I wrote mentioning him. It seems I may have upset him.'

'I will see if he is in his office and available to talk. Please hold the line.'

A few minutes went by as I waited for the knight to pick up the telephone.

'Sir John Smith here! Peter McDonald? Ah yes, the column in Hospital Doctor? Yes, yes. My son, who is a doctor in London and reads your column regularly, sent me a copy of your piece. Very accurate and really rather amusing. Absolutely no need to apologise. Good day to you.'

Suddenly the sun was shining and a great weight had been lifted off my shoulders. I had been lucky that the good chairman had a sense of humour. A man in authority who was happy to attract sturdy debate. Not pusillanimous as some senior managers and consultants can be.

I wrote a note to the senior consultant at Southampton relating the gist of my telephone conversation with the chairman. I knew that would be the end of the affair and that he, the bombast, had been made to look rather petty.

It had been an uncomfortable episode and it had caused me substantial grief. Trying to make my readers smile when they read my pieces can be costly indeed.

But in this case, I can truthfully say I enjoyed the last laugh.

***

Over the years that I have written opinion articles I have had many such close scrapes. Late one evening after a tot of Famous Grouse, I remember writing that the worst surgeon that I had ever worked with, was now a professor of surgery. Within a week three professors had written threatening to sue me. One of them was right but I was not going to divulge to them which one it was.

At least, my own professor knew, from the way I had expressed myself in the article, it was not to him I was referring. However, he took me aside a day or two later.

'Peter, don't you think it is time to put up your journalistic pen and concentrate on writing more surgical papers? I know you are doing fairly well but these articles are distracting you from these efforts.'

Of course, he was right and I should have thrown away my ballpoint and Amstrad computer there and then. But I could not. Like many scribblers you cannot stop. It is a sort of obsession. Like gambling or alcohol, it is hard to desist. The result was that my column was rebranded the next week and I carried on writing under the nom de plume 'Dr. Slop'. This was the name of the bad-tempered man-midwife in Tristram Shandy's Sentimental Journey and his name seemed to chime with my character. Certainly, my wife

Christina uses it as a gentle tease on a weekly basis though I cannot imagine why.

For a year Dr. Slop wrote about the imaginary Midhampton General Hospital which led to me writing the novel A Trust in Conflict a few years later. But even Dr. Slop was not immune to gaffs. In the final episode of the story published more than a year later the hero, a consultant surgeon, was described secretly filming the trust's chief executive chasing a tart around a hotel bedroom. Something to blackmail him with, perhaps?

In A Trust in Conflict the chief executive is corrupt and needed to be removed by fair means or foul. Nothing particularly salacious about that but the magazine's cartoonist got carried away by the piece. Normally cartoonists embellish an article but, on this occasion, he nearly finished off my writing career.

He depicted a full-chested near-naked lady being chased around the room by an old man who seemed only to be wearing a pair of socks. Both the editor, who published it, and I thought it was very funny reflecting my vision for the characters. But the Managing Editor of Hospital Doctor had a different opinion and was not a happy with what he considered quasi-pornographic.

The week after the cartoon was published the editor telephoned me.

'Peter, I am afraid my boss is disgusted with Dr. Slop and has told me to cut your column. It is a case of, if you don't go, I do!'

I was pretty sure I knew what the outcome would be so I pre-empted the harassed editor before he had time to continue.

'OK Nigel, I could just come back under my own name next week? It's been a year since that business with the three professors.'

'Alright Peter. Back to basics. Slop and Midhampton are mincemeat but it was good fun while it lasted. Look forward to your copy under your own name on Monday.'

And so, my column gained a new lease of life and I continued writing for Hospital Doctor for another decade until that periodical died. It ran out of money when government legislation on pharmaceutical advertising meant Big Pharma could no longer support free-to-read publications for doctors.

Much later John Black, a man with a special sense of humour and a much admired President of the Royal College of England, of which I am a fellow, asked me to write a column for The Bulletin, their in-house news and information journal. With a readership of 25,000 I would have been mad not to take up the challenge. I created, for a small monthly stipend, a new character, 'Mr. Slop FRCS'. A harassed, aging surgeon living under the shadow of Mount Middle in the heart of England is set upon on a monthly basis by his Esteemed Editors to write whatever they decree whether he knows something or nothing of it. Another chance for the scribbler to vent his spleen.

With Mr. Slop now past his centenary column, he has become an institution of sorts leavening the serious business of British surgery in the twenty-first century. One day I suppose he will run out of surgical steam and I will be sad when Mr. Slop reaches the age of senility, or forgets how to hit 'send' on his Apple Mac.

Other columns have come and gone. For twenty years I was 'Gemellus', as I am an identical twin, for a serious journal called Colorectal Disease. It was a column where I was paid well to read the literature I was supposed to be reading anyway. I would comment about it in a colourful way. What could be better? I learnt a few things from writing it. In recent years I have been struck how the research output coming from Korea and China has been growing fast while it has been diminishing from the US and the UK. Asian flowers are obviously blooming even in my obscure branch of surgery.

Gemellus had quite a following but he died suddenly when a new editor was appointed. So Gemellus went the way of all literary flesh.

Writers hate change. When editors come and go so do we. We have no control. We are always vulnerable. We are ships passing in the night. A columnist's job is to write provocatively and then disappear.

My guess is that sadly too, we are quickly forgotten.

***

But if columns come and go so other opportunities arise. Two decades ago, I published The Oxford Dictionary of Medical Quotations with the Oxford University Press. We sold a couple of thousand hardbacks and some five thousand paperbacks but then it fizzled out. It was a lot of effort but great fun.

Being an opportunist, I sent a copy of the book and a cheeky letter to Nigel Rees, the creator of the long-running quiz programme Quote/Unquote on BBC Radio Four. I suggested I might be one of his guests on his show. He kindly took up my offer and I appeared on six of his shows with other minor celebrities such as the late William Franklin, 'the voice', the recently deceased John Sessions, the actor, and even Michael (Lord) Grade, the media executive. This led to other opportunities, reasonable fees and lots more fun.

But for me as a serious surgeon it was just that. Lots of fun. But for the actors it was their life. I remember being reminded more than once by Jeremy Beadle and others that I had a real and important job while their careers they felt were sometimes devoid of depth and meaning. Frivolous, insecure, not truly important. It was an interesting slant on their lives and one which rang true.

As I met more show business types, there did, indeed, seem to be a void in their souls that only fooling around could hide. This has been said of comedians before but it probably could be applied to thespians of all shades. I have seen it in bankers too, when the motive of money wears thin.

When I left the sets of BBC Radio Four I went back to my day job, saving lives and relieving pain, while they went home to hope their agent phoned with more work of a frivolous nature. A contrast, indeed.

**

I have not met many other doctors who have the scribbling gene although I have been on a podium with Henry Marsh, the neurosurgeon, who has had great success with First Do No Harm. But scribbling, like an itchy bottom, never quite goes away. It is not something you can ever truly hide. But when I discover it in a fellow medical traveller, I find I have a lot in common with them.

My registrar Nick Taffinder had the gene. Once we learnt that we suffered from the same affliction we knew we would be friends. He had that entrepreneurial inquisitiveness that is the trait of any writer and quickly I put him to good use. We started a new weekly column together and managed to persuade an editor to publish it. One week he would write it and the next I would. A shared experience and a good discipline. It was a review column called Avicenna (AD 980 - 1037) named after the great physician, philosopher of the Persian School of medicine.

For a year we wrote this column together and then started work on another paper on high-street colonic irrigation, or hydrotherapy, which was eventually published in the respectable Colorectal Disease journal. Like me Nick had an unconventional approach to our profession so when I suggested we look into this odd lay activity he jumped at the idea. Coming from the mistaken assumption that faeces stuck in the colon must be harmful to health, the aficionados of colonic hydrotherapy pay good money to have it all washed out from below. A kind of emptying of a sluice.

I had the notion that we might document what the patients and the colonic hydrotherapy practitioners believed to be the benefits of this untested treatment. I supposed the practice had developed from the concept of enemas that have been used for millennia. The ancient Egyptians certainly employed enemas to infuse medicaments or to empty the bowels. Presumably, like today's hydrotherapy punters, they felt better for it but we will never know because they are just mummies now.

Nick organised the research with enthusiasm and was invited to lecture to the annual meeting of the Association of Colonic Hydrotherapists to talk about it. Handing out questionnaires at the meeting quickly brought in the data and the paper took shape. I would present our results a year later to the same meeting.

At one point in the research, it was clear that one of us should experience what colonic irrigation was in order to write about it.

'Peter, you know I am a better photographer than you. I will film you having the enema for the project,' he joked.

'But...?' I protested.

'Fine...that's agreed then!'

Nick was a charming and persuasive man so I had little option but to concur. He was right. I am a lousy photographer. A few weeks later I found myself on the table of an irrigation room in Harley Street in the hands of a practitioner who was said to have regularly irrigated a royal personage. Then began a series of washouts up a proctoscope, an instrument that goes into the anus, with the hydrotherapist describing, in unnecessary detail, the exact nature of the effluent emerging from my rear end. It was both amusing and embarrassing as Nick clicked away with his camera but it provided us good pictures for subsequent lectures.

The paper was well received and Nick soon left to take up his consultant post. As testament as to how I thought about Nick, I enrolled him into my surgical travelling club, The Needles, of which I was a founder member. I hoped our productive professional and personal relationship would last for many years to come.

How cruelly mistaken this aspiration would turn out to be.

In Kent, where Nick had become a consultant, he was seen as a brilliant surgeon and had very quickly built a flourishing practice. One day a couple of years later he developed back pain which somehow would not go away. After six weeks he persuaded one of his radiological colleagues to take an X-ray of his back and pelvis. It was duly reported as normal.

Relieved but still confused as to the origin of the pain he took the X-ray home and showed it to Jane, his wife then looking after their four children. She was a trained physiotherapist specialising in respiratory care often reading chest X-rays but rarely pelvic or spinal ones. As she peered at the X-ray held up to the morning light, she was puzzled.

'Nick, why is it all white on this side of the pelvis and dark on the other?'

'Well, it is because…?'

Nick halted with his explanation as he suddenly realised, for the first time, the obvious asymmetry on the X-ray. The left side of the pelvis, where his pain was centred, was opaque while the right clear. The difference was so marked that both he and his colleague the radiologist had assumed it was an artifact, a shadow caused in the taking of the X-ray by some external technical factor.

But they were both wrong. It was a monster hiding in plain sight.

A dense tumour projects white and opaque on an X-ray. Ordinary soft tissue is darker.

Tragically for this married couple Jane's observation was the start of a two-and-a-half-year ordeal that would have no happy ending.

In the next few days, a CT scan, a biopsy and an orthopaedic opinion confirmed that Nick had a very large histiocytoma, a malignant bone tumour, arising from the left side of his pelvis. There was evidence of spread to his chest too. It would mean very specialised treatment and the chance of success was very low.

I know little of the details of Nick's treatment except the fact that a few months later he was in the Royal National Orthopaedic Hospital, Stanmore having a procedure to support his now partially removed pelvis. It was the evening before he was to undergo another operation when the charge nurse on duty that night entered his side room.

'Nick, I know you are a colorectal surgeon but I hope you don't mind me asking you a few questions on my behalf.'

'Please do,' replied Nick always keen to help others.

'Well, I've had this rectal bleeding and the feeling I need to go all the time to the loo almost as if there is something stuck there.'

Nick had heard this story a dozen times before and it usually did not end well.

'Look Liam I do not like the sound of this. To cut the red tape the best thing would be to allow me to do a rectal examination. Now.'

Both men knew that this was logical but almost without precedent. A patient metamorphosing into the doctor and the nurse looking after him becoming the patient? Not conventional behaviour but needs must. For Nick there was probably a life at stake that evening at Stanmore and this time it was not his.

So, in the middle night the colorectal surgeon, awaiting an orthopaedic procedure for a life-threatening problem, performed a rectal examination on the nurse who was looking after him. By anyone's measure this was an act of not only of extreme compassion but also of courage.

It only took a minute or two for the surgeon to get the information he needed.

Nick did not like at all what he could feel through the Latex glove. A hard mass typical of a rectal cancer. Being in no position to help Liam himself, he decided to phone his old boss, now his friend.

***

It was 6.30am that next morning and I was driving on my way to work when I got the call from Nick.

'Hi mate! How's the treatment going?' I joked trying to sound upbeat about Nick's predicament.

'Peter, I need your help,' replied Nick who I knew was currently an inpatient at Stanmore.

When I had heard the story I instructed him to tell Liam to be in my outpatients at St. Mark's at 10am and I would see him personally.

'Thanks Peter. See you soon.'

Liam came to see me that morning and I confirmed Nick's findings. After investigations had diagnosed a cancer of the rectum, three weeks later I performed an abdomino-perineal resection leaving him with a permanent colostomy. It was a standard but very major operation for a low rectal cancer. I removed his rectum and anus to prevent the cancer from spreading. Post-operatively he underwent a course of chemotherapy and, to this day, he is well, retired from active nursing practice, and living in Spain.

There is no question in my mind that Nick's actions that night at Stanmore probably saved Liam's life. However inappropriate it might seem for the patient to assume the role of the doctor, he was right to do just that. If he had not done so it could have been several months before Liam had arranged to see his GP and get access to the help he needed. By then the tumour might just have been out of control and incurable. Who knows?

A few months later Nick, knowing his own battle with cancer was being lost, wrote a Personal View for the British Medical Journal and it contained an account of that extraordinary night in the orthopaedic ward. It was one of the most moving pieces of medical writing I have ever read.

The reaction to Nick's article was both shocking and interesting. In the letter section of the journal some small-minded doctors thought he had overstepped the mark and that his actions were unethical. I judge that these are doctors who are unable to see the bigger picture. They are fixated on protocol unable to cut through the red tape that often hampers our lives. Quite simply these constraints are to be ignored when there is a greater need outwith these conventions. Instead of censuring Nick they should have applauded the bravery of a dying man who overstepped an artificial barrier in order to serve another.

***

The next few months were hard for Nick. More chemotherapy at the Royal Marsden Hospital and a few more stabilising operations followed. My last meeting with Nick was when I visited him on the ward there.

'Hi Nick you are not looking too bad,' I said, lying but trying to bolster his confidence.

'Peter I feel rough. It is not going that well I'm afraid. Can you take me out to the Indian restaurant round the corner and we can eat a hot curry and drink a pint of lager?'

'But is that allowed?' I asked knowing too well the answer.

'No, certainly it is not. But no-one will notice us sneaking out.'

I needed no more persuasion so together we slid quietly past the nurses' office while they were doing their evening handovers.

The tasty meal we shared that night was my last supper with Nick. This bold, talented, young surgeon died eight weeks later surrounded by the family that loved him dearly.

He was a truly remarkable man and it was not fair that Fate had singled him out for an early death. At his funeral service there were hundreds packed into the little country church in Kent mourning his passing and grieving their loss.

I had not wept so many tears since I lost my own father and mother.

***

I started this chapter by writing about journalism and I finished it with a description of the death of a fine surgeon who could write well.

I make no apology for that lack of alignment except that it tells two stories that are inextricably linked.

Courage to stick one's neck out on the page on the one hand, and courage by Nick to do the right thing for Liam, the nurse who became his patient, on the other.

RIP Mr. Nicholas Taffinder MBBS MS FRCS.

***

Nick's bravery was self-evident but he was rewarded cruelly by dying before his time. Other patients I have treated have been equally plucky in adversity but, by dint of fortune, have not been dealt such a bad hand. I remember one whose misfortune began the day I first clapped eyes on him.

It began with a stroll through the X-ray Department one busy lunchtime…

Chapter 12:
How My Patient Was Front Page News

❖

I remember that Friday morning in 1992 quite clearly. I had finished my outpatient clinic and was rushing to review the X-rays of a patient under my care. I had operated that Tuesday on a tumour in the oesophagus and the patient had an unexplained fever and I was worried about him. Although he did not have a great deal of continuing pain, I felt it was important to get a quick contrast study to see if my anastomosis, or join-up, had leaked.

Earlier that morning my patient had been wheeled down to the Imaging Department and swallowed some radio-opaque dye called gastrografin to see if everything was in order. Not a task that either the patient or the radiologist like much but if it was normal it would allow me to sleep that night.

My radiological colleague Bob reassured me in his small, dark office that all was hunky dory with the new gullet I had fashioned, bringing up the stomach into the chest. By demonstrating that my handiwork was intact, he greatly relieved my anxiety. With nothing else on the scan to worry us, I knew that this patient would be ready for discharge in four or five days and thankfully I would not have to spend the evening in theatre sorting out the problem.

Little did I know then that I was not going to get much rest that night at all, for a completely different reason.

Much relieved I was heading to the canteen to get a quick bite to eat before going off to do a theatre list at another hospital.

It was on my way out of the Imaging Department that I spotted Mr. Baker.

A large fellow, he was lying on a bed in the main X-ray corridor outside the new CT scanner. He was propped high up on pillows. He did not look a good colour and he had a very worried expression on his lop-sided face. The reason for the asymmetry was because of a huge swelling expanding from the right side of his neck. Although it was not quite my area of interest, I wondered if it might be a nasty tonsillar abscess. I knew from my medical student days these abscesses can get really big and need incising urgently to let the pus out. Perhaps he had some additional spreading cellulitis or bacterial infection that they were worried about so wanted a scan? I could see from the name on the end of the bed he was under the care of one our ear, nose and throat (ENT) consultants.

I smiled at the gentleman warmly as he had caught my inquisitive eye.

Just as I did so he moved a little in his bed and the flimsy gauze dressing, which was very loosely taped over the swelling, shifted a little. Under it I could see the lump more clearly, and to my horror, just below its most protuberant part, was a grey-black patch of gangrenous skin the size of a small saucer. To me this meant only one thing.

Necrotising fasciitis, or spreading dermal gangrene. Once skin gangrene is visible I knew that the infection could not be brought under control without radical and potentially mutilating surgery. The treatment is to remove all dead tissue. In that instant of passing him in the corridor I had no doubt that without immediate surgery this patient would not survive. In addition, I knew the overall mortality from this most feared condition was more than 30% even with appropriate surgical debridement.

It was a clear case of what later in the same decade became known popularly as the 'flesh-eating bug'.

Being careful to disguise my growing alarm, I stopped to talk to him for a few minutes. I quickly learnt a little more about his predicament. He was a taxi-driver. Sixty-years old and a late-onset diabetic who had been suffering with pain and swelling in his neck for about five days. He told me wearily that he was not getting better despite antibiotics. Now he felt awful.

'Do you know Mr. Dhillon, the ENT surgeon, looking after me? 'He's a very kind doctor,' he added.

'Yes, I know Mr. Dhillon quite well. I might give him a ring because I think there might be some useful advice I can give him.'

I decided to delay my afternoon theatre list for an hour and went back to my office and telephoned him.

'Hi there Ram? Peter McDonald here. We have met once or twice in the coffee room but never more than that, I believe. I am phoning about Mr. Baker your patient. I hope you don't mind me interfering but I came across him in the Imaging Department and he appears to have necrotising fasciitis. He has a patch of gangrene with all the other features of a spreading synergistic infection. I think he needs it all excised very urgently if he is to survive.'

'Gosh, Peter. I have never seen that condition before. I remember reading about it in my training. In our specialty it is almost unheard of. I suppose the blood supply at our end is so good we are spared it. As far as I know it has hardly ever been described in the head and neck region. Are you sure it is necrotising fasciitis?'

'Yes, I am certain. We see it a lot below the belt particularly around the anus and scrotum so we are more on the look-out for it than you lot would be. But this chap needs surgery immediately if he is going to survive. If you like I can come and see him formally with you now and then help you in theatre tonight? I think the infection is spreading down the chest wall outside your territory so you will probably need a general surgeon like me anyway.'

Ram, who was a bit shocked by what I had told him, seemed grateful that I had brought this to his attention. He agreed that we should look after the patient together. We saw him within a half hour, explained the sudden change of plan and got his agreement for the operation.

So began a surgical journey that would start around dinner time and continue into the early hours. It would necessitate a lengthy period in the Intensive Care Unit and extensive plastic reconstructive surgery at a later date. En route, Mr. Baker would be close to death but he would become an instant celebrity with his face on the front of a tabloid newspaper.

Later that day Mr. Baker, whose blood pressure was now sagging, was consented, prepped and ready to be anaesthetised. I remember trying to cheer him up but when we consented him I was forced to make it plain to him that he was going to wake up greatly disfigured. I explained that it was the only way his life could be saved. He was stunned, but like most London taxi drivers, he was a brave, solid sort.

This kind of information is never an easy thing to impart to a patient. It is a part of my job I have always hated. But it has to be done honestly but tinged with a heavy dose of optimism. Patients often forget later the pains they suffer in the course of their treatments but they always remember the words we use when we consent them. They remember even more the tone of our speech. It is from these often brief moments of contact between the doctors and their patients that the label of a good or bad bedside manner is earned.

Necrotising fasciitis, idiopathic or synergistic gangrene is a mouthful of nasty, frightening sounding words. It is enough to confuse anyone whether they are in the medical profession or outside. First described by Jean Fournier in Paris in the nineteenth century and defined more fully in 1933 by Frank Meleney, professor of surgery in Columbia, New York, it is a condition that strikes terror into the hearts of surgeons for they know that, even in the era of antibiotics that are effective for many conditions, watching and waiting is not an option.

This is compounded by the fact it is very difficult to diagnose. On the one hand patients are treated later than ideal because in the early stages of the condition there is no black, gangrenous tissue visible. It is probable on the other hand that other patients are subjected to unnecessary surgery for fear of missing the condition. Surgeons are damned if they do and damned if they hesitate.

Like any successful campaign of war amongst allies, a mixture of pathogenic bacteria join forces together to defeat the human host. Coliforms, staphylococci, bacteroides species, anaerobic streptococci and peptostreptococci to name a few. Antibiotics cannot penetrate dead tissue when the blood supply is lost. The condition rapidly causes systemic infection and multi-organ failure if not treated.

Sepsis. A word now familiar to many today. Skin, fat, fascia and muscle all eventually lose their blood supply and die. Only surgical excision seems able to stop the literal rot that overwhelms the patient.

Surgery entails cutting out all dead tissue wherever it lies. If that means sacrificing large areas of soft tissue, so be it. Thankfully necrotising fasciitis hardly ever enters the body cavities and never involves bone. Essential internal structures are almost always spared. That does not mean the patient is off the hook. All the hard, dead fat and non-bleeding muscle, not just the gangrenous or grey-black part, must be removed. This means the patient may lose vast areas of soft tissue. In certain areas of the body this can be hidden and is just a painful inconvenience but in other parts, such as the face, this is a disaster.

I had treated this fearful condition a dozen times before, mostly in the region of the anus, buttocks, abdominal wall, scrotum and groins, for which it appears to have a particular affinity. I have had to remove great slices of tissue from the abdomen. Excising the scrotum leaving the testicles uncovered and unprotected is a particular horror. However, like Ram Dhillon, I had never seen it above the nipples until that day and certainly not on the face or neck. Although it was clear in my mind what had to be done to Mr. Baker, there is always a little grain of uncertainty as to whether I was doing the right thing at exactly the right moment.

As the surgery got underway Ram began tentatively cutting away the grey-black carapace on Mr. Baker's neck. I was forced to urge him to expand his area of excision as he extirpated larger and larger areas of lifeless fat and muscle in the neck. I was relieved, as expected, that the major neck veins and arteries, the jugulars, the carotids and the vertebral arteries were spared. Eventually Ram was burrowing around at the base of the skull getting close to structures that I, a general and bowel surgeon, had last seen or read about in my anatomy vivas for the Royal College of Surgeons' examinations.

It was all very scary.

There was grey fluid oozing out between the muscles attached to the base of the skull and much more tissue than expected had to be removed. I could see Ram Dhillon was getting very nervous, almost alarmed.

'Cut away Ram, we have no choice. All the dead stuff must come out. If there is any doubt we can leave the areas we are uncertain about and come back in forty-eight hours. But experience has shown that the more radical we are on the first sitting the more likely he will survive.'

'OK, Peter if you are sure?'

'Quite sure,' I confirmed.

With a lowish blood pressure from the worsening sepsis, I had judged Mr. Baker's chances of survival before we started at less than 50%. I knew we had to remove all we possibly could. After a couple of hours Ram, who was sweating visibly under the hot lights of the operating theatre, had finished removing all dead tissue in the head and neck. That was his region of expertise though he had never had to do anything quite like this before.

It was now my turn as the general surgeon to go below the neck area and continue the life-saving mutilation.

'Let's see how far this bloody thing goes down on his chest wall,' I said.

I then sliced off sliver after sliver of dead skin and fat from the lower edge of Ram's wound. I progressed bit by bit over Mr. Baker's right shoulder and right pectoral area. By the time I reached healthy bleeding tissue and muscle I had been forced to remove half of the sternomastoid, deltoid and pectoralis major muscles as well as his right nipple and some of the latissimus dorsi muscle. At the end of the operation, we had a wound the size of three dinner plates with just a few small living muscles, such as the scalenes, covering the vital nerves and vessels in his neck.

It was not a sight for the faint-hearted. The patient had lost about six units of blood and lots of serum in the process. It was still very oozy and we then had to spend twenty minutes getting the bleeding under control. Then we packed into the wound layers of gauze dressings and Gamgee, the latter a time-honoured absorbent cotton layer between the gauze, named after a British 19th Century surgeon.

Nowadays we might use a more modern dressing but in the early nineties we were still using traditional ones.

By two o'clock in the morning the job was done and Mr. Baker was shipped to the intensive care unit where the intensivists planned to ventilate him for as long as would be needed. They continued to infuse blood, other intravenous fluids, broad-spectrum antibiotics and inotropes, cardiac supporting drugs, to keep him alive.

I remember climbing into my bed in Hertfordshire at three in the morning utterly exhausted but certain we had done the right thing for Ram's patient.

The next few days were critical for Mr. Baker but, despite his diabetes and huge oozing wound, it soon became clear to me that he had enough reserve capacity to fight this lethal concoction of hostile bacteria. We took him back to theatre twice over that long weekend to inspect and redress the wound. We were forced to remove further small areas of necrotic tissue that we had left behind that had no blood supply. But overall, the wound was looking good and we were heartened by his progress.

By the fifth day he came off the ventilator and the intensivists began to wean him off the strong medicines. He could now communicate but not talk. He smiled lopsidedly to me and I imagined that he winked at me with his good eye.

He would survive.

By the time he got back onto the main surgical ward a week later he was no longer in danger. What was needed now was a period of daily dressings under the joint care of our visiting plastic surgeon. These were extensive and painful. It was hard for Mr. Baker as he returned to full consciousness. He understood properly for the first time what we had been forced to do to him. I hoped no-one would offer him a mirror to look into but if they did I judged that he was ready for the shock that would follow.

But he was a fighter with the wicked sense of humour of a born and bred Londoner. Once I had appreciated this I knew he would be psychologically resilient in the long term. Certainly, he would need to be very stoical and patient as he had a long way to go before he would be physically and mentally healed.

After three weeks he was transferred to Mount Vernon Hospital and the plastic surgeons took over responsibility for him. I lost touch with him but he was still in my mind as Ram and I wrote up his case for publication. As it was one of the few reported cases of necrotising fasciitis of the head and neck in the world literature, we published it in the Journal of Laryngology and Otology as Cervical Necrotising Fasciitis and Tonsilitis. Not a journal I was ever in the habit of reading, or publishing research in, but the article was well received by ENT surgeons around the world.

I like to think it may have helped some make the diagnosis of necrotising fasciitis quicker than they would otherwise have done.

If that was the case more than just a few lives would have been saved.

***

In the next few months Mr. Baker had to undergo a series of four reconstructive plastic operations. One day that summer he sent me a picture of his reconstructed face and neck. Although not an adonis before his illness, the final cosmetic was remarkably pleasing. The plastic surgeons had excelled themselves. With his permission I kept this image for lectures to students and young surgeons and showed it as often as I could.

But that was not the end of Mr. Baker's story of misery and redemption. Two years after we had operated upon him a gentleman of the press wrote an article about the condition of necrotising fasciitis or spreading gangrene. The piece suggested it was a new disease that the doctors were powerless to treat. In good journalistic mode the resourceful hack decided to popularise his discovery. The public panicked and the story of rogue bacterias spread around the world. In fact, surgeons had known all about it for one hundred and fifty years. But who worries about accuracy when there is a good story to write? As a scribbler myself, I cannot be overcritical.

Accounts of an epidemic in Gloucestershire circulated as five patients with necrotising fasciitis were reported in that area in a short period of time. In the end it was concluded that this was just a random cluster of cases as no connection could be made between them. Although Mr. Baker, as far as I know, had never been to Gloucestershire in his taxi, he managed to climb on the band-wagon and sold his story to the press. Labelled KILLER BUG ATE MY FACE at least one tabloid, the Daily Star went to town.

His cheeky, smiling, newly-reconstructed face stared at me from the front page of that newspaper one morning. I was quoted as telling him that:

'Your only chance is that we cut away your face, neck and chest. It's rotten flesh and we must take it away immediately.'

The story of that night was dramatically retold. It explained how he was given a Phantom of The Opera style mask so his visitors would not get so upset.

A few weeks after his story hit the front page, he sent me a copy of the original picture and a second note of thanks attached to a bottle of malt whisky. This was a case of a man making good in adversity. I greatly admired his ingenuity in grasping the opportunity to sell his story even though the science expressed was greatly suspect.

Good for Mr. Baker. Brave fellow. I hope they paid him handsomely.

The thirst for medical stories seems unquenchable. I suppose it has always been that way. Humans like to be scared. It stimulates their anxious juices and gives them that odd bitter/sweet sensation of there-but-for-the-Grace-of-God-go-I. Stories of terrible diseases are reported widely. Journalists re-discover on a daily basis rare conditions that have been known about for centuries. Doctors are forced to remind correspondents sometimes that there really is not very much new under the medical sun.

But new threats do emerge from time to time. Other diseases disappear from human consciousness. Memories are short. Few today remember that Frère Jacques Beaulieu (1651-1720), after who the nursery rhyme was written, was a travelling surgical lithotomist and a Dominican Friar. A man with a scant knowledge of anatomy who cut for bladder stones often with fatal consequences. The song calls for the bells of matins to be rung to rouse Frère Jacques who has apparently overslept. He was kept very busy because bladder stones were very common in the Middle Ages but have practically disappeared today.

Pre-dating the good friar by three hundred years was the scourge of The Black Death and pandemics which we will meet again in a later chapter. HIV and AIDS, Mad Cow Disease, Ebola, SARS, MERS and Covid-19 are, of course, new diseases that have had no true equivalents in history and when they emerge as new epidemics the penny drops quite slowly that a new disease has arrived.

New diseases are fascinating to learn about but disquieting at the same time. I was already a surgical registrar when I first heard the term HIV, or human immunodeficiency syndrome. It was uncomfortable to learn about a disease while being in the front line instead of in a lecture hall at medical school. We all made many wrong assumptions. We believed it was highly infectious and would soon overwhelm the NHS. I remember visualising a huge HIV tower block being built beside every general hospital in the land. I thought it would dominate modern medicine and I even advised my young house officers to consider specialising in this new disease. We believed it to be confined to one group, MSM, as it is now called – Men who have Sex with Men.

We were wrong.

We thought the condition would never be brought under control and that it would never be cured. We were wrong on the first count and soon, it seems likely, we may be proved wrong on the second.

New diseases appear when least expected. Doctors and journalists must stand ready to describe the new syndromes when they arise but be always aware that they may be peddling old stories too as in the case of the necrotising fasciitis and the flesh-eating bugs.

For Mr. Baker and his neck abscess this mattered not at all. He got the treatment he needed and, indirectly, he helped to enlarge the world's medical literature and thus increase the world's awareness of a condition and to help them to be even more vigilant in future.

And hopefully he was paid well for his one day of fame. It would have been a small but well-deserved compensation for his unlucky ordeal and the mutilation we had to inflict on him that night to save his life.

But it is not only the patient who suffers when disease strikes as we will see in the next chapter.

Chapter 13:
A Brace Of Victims

❖

William came to see me one Tuesday morning at my St. Mark's outpatient clinic. He had attended his GP the week before when he had noticed some rectal bleeding. It had started a couple of months previously but he had delayed a few weeks to get to see the doctor. The blood from his back passage had been mixed with his stool and, as the weeks wore on, he had the feeling of something needing to be passed but it would not come out. This symptom goes by the unusual word tenesmus (from the Greek teinesmos – a stretching). Although it may have a harmless cause at times, it is quite often associated with a space occupying lesion, or tumour, in the rectum.

When William mentioned this symptom to me my interest and fears were immediately aroused. Most patients who have overt rectal bleeding are suffering from haemorrhoids or an anal fissure. Something rather painful and inconvenient but not worrying. But if they are bleeding and, at the same time, complain of tenesmus they are more likely to have significant trouble. After hearing the story, I advised William that I needed to perform a rectal examination and a sigmoidoscopy.

Digital examination of the rectum is an undignified procedure for both patient and doctor but yields a great deal of information. A patient asked me recently how often I had carried it out and did I know how unpleasant it was. I replied that I did know what a miserable business it could be and that I had performed it about sixty-thousand times on well over a third of the one hundred and fifty-thousand patients I had treated over five decades. The patient seemed relieved that they had not been singled out for special treatment.

As a veteran rectal examiner, I am grateful that I have been fortunate to practise my proctological trade in the era of rubber or latex disposable gloves. My predecessors were forced to do it bare-fingered with just some soap under their fingernail. In 1894 William Halsted, a professor of surgery at Johns Hopkins Hospital, Baltimore developed rubber gloves primarily for protection against dermatitis but it was not until 1964 that the disposable rubber glove became widely available.

Back to my outpatient clinic.

I turned William on his left side and placed my well-lubricated, gloved, index finger into his rectum. It took no more than a second to know that my worst fears had been realised. The hardness of the rectal cancer in the lower rectum was immediately obvious. Ulcerated in the middle with raised edges I had felt this monster too many times before. At least this one was not fixed to the pelvic side walls. It was quite mobile. Thinking ahead, I knew it would not be too difficult to remove when the time came.

I passed a sigmoidoscope and took a couple of big biopsies and put them in formalin in a pot.

After I had finished and the patient was dressed we talked. William had his wife with him. I judged they were a together couple who would be able to support each other through the hard times to come.

'What's the trouble, doctor?' he asked quietly.

I could see how worried he was.

'Well, although I cannot say for certain until the biopsy is back, I think you have a cancer of the rectum William.'

'Oh dear! Does that mean an operation?'

'It means you are at the beginning of a long journey which will need more investigations and then, perhaps, an operation. I do not think you will need radiotherapy but probably some post-operative chemotherapy to soak up any cells around the body once the tumour is out.'

'That sounds bad!'

'Well, it is and it isn't. The tumour seems confined to the rectum and is both mobile and high enough for me to join you up and put your plumbing back together. It might mean a temporary stoma or bag but we should be able to close it a few weeks after the operation.'

The next fifteen minutes was spent going over some of these details before I passed him on to one of our MacMillan Cancer Nurse Specialists to go through it again in much greater detail. Without intending, we doctors and nurses have created a classic bad cop/good cop routine which works rather well. As a surgeon (the bad cop) my role is to deliver the unpleasant news while our highly skilled nurse (the good cop), oozing sympathy, reassures and fills in the gaps in the patient's understanding.

It adds another twenty minutes to the consultation but allows me to see another patient in an adjacent room. These first encounters are so vital if the ground work of good care is to be laid down well. More importantly the patients and their relatives will remember those first few minutes with us more than any other time under our care. Every word said and every expression used is imprinted in their minds.

At the end of the briefing, they were reassured that they would be able to cope and, when William and his wife finally left the outpatients an hour later, I could hear them talking quite happily together. It was almost as if the Sword of Damocles I had held above them was a fantasy of my own imagination.

***

William came in for his cancer operation four weeks later. In the meantime, he had undergone a colonoscopy, chest X-ray, ultrasound of the liver and some blood tests. This was in the days before we had access to routine CT even though the first CT machine in the world was actually tested in our hospital, Northwick Park, in 1975.

The operation I had planned for him was an anterior resection of the rectum, so called as it was performed through an abdominal incision from the front. Until the First World War all operations on the rectum for tumours were carried out by a posterior approach by incising alongside the sacrum. It was deemed too dangerous to work from the front as it would be inside the peritoneal cavity, the fear of peritonitis before the advent of antibiotics being so great.

After the Second World War surgeons were emboldened to go in from the front led by a pioneering surgeon called Claude Dixon in the USA and much later by my old boss Bill Heald from Basingstoke, who popularised the use of mechanical stapling devices and an ultra-precise dissection of the pelvic structures. Apart from the innovation of laparoscopic and minimally invasive surgery and now the robotic machines that aid this method, this is still the modern approach.

With the patient paralysed and anaesthetised, I made a midline incision in the abdomen. I mobilised the rectum down to the pelvic floor and divided it above the next part of the colon, the sigmoid colon, and brought the left side of the colon down and joined it up to the remaining rectal stump deep in the pelvis. I employed a circular stapling gun to effect this and I was happy with the result.

No tension and a good blood supply.

Although these operations were done for years by placing a large number of sutures, nowadays the staple guns speed up the process and are a great help when access is difficult. First developed in Russia, the Americans subsequently stole the show with their well-engineered, disposable, single-use devices.

I was greatly relieved that there was no sign of spread of the tumour outside the rectum. The lymph nodes near the rectum were not obviously involved either. This meant that William had about a 60% chance of complete cure. With a bit of adjuvant chemotherapy that figure might even rise to 70%.

Although the operation had gone without a hitch, I formed a temporary loop ileostomy in the lower right side of the abdomen. This is an opening on the surface of the abdomen into the last part of the small intestine. This would allow the litre of small bowel effluent to be collected in a bag and avoid it going through the join-up. This would greatly reduce the consequences of a leak if it happened. Despite all our best efforts, a leak occurs, for reasons not often clear, in about 10% of cases. It is often a very serious complication and needs to be managed well if the patient is not to succumb.

Post-operatively William initially did very well. He was mobilising on the ward and his bowels were beginning to work as the ileostomy bag began to fill. He was over the worst of the pain and was feeling pretty confident. He was pleased to receive the news from my resident surgical officer that the tumour had been confined to his pelvis.

In the first four days his recovery was therefore as good as could be hoped for.

***

I wish I could have said that my own recovery from his four hour operation was the same. The day after the procedure I started to ache all over. My muscles screamed to me that I had run a marathon. That evening I had a rigor and a high temperature. I shook and sweated, on and off, most of the night. The coughing started the following day and by the third day I could hardly get out of bed. This was not just a cold. It had to be influenza.

It was the worst I had felt for years.

I telephoned my assistant and explained the difficulty.

'Keep an eye on William in particular. If you have any problems with any of the patients get Professor Munro to see them for me. I think I am going to have to lie low and sweat this one out.'

The next three days were not easy.

In my life I have been very lucky in avoiding serious illness only having needed to take a week or two off work in more than fifty years. Although I had my tonsils out as a child under ether, I have never since even had an injection for pain. Indeed, when I am performing colonoscopies and gastroscopies, I joke with my patients, as I administer pethidine or fentanyl to them and they drift into the opioid bliss that follows, that I have yet to experience the wondrous but addictive feelings that these euphoric drugs create.

By the weekend I felt even worse. It was clear I was in for the long-haul. At the same time, I received a message that William was not doing so well and that Professor Munro had been up to see him. He thought he might have a limited leak from my join-up. An urgent CT was arranged but did not confirm one or offer any other clue to explain his fever, fast pulse and severe fatigue.

No urinary tract infection.

No deep vein thrombosis.

His chest was clear.

His heart sound.

Over that weekend I fretted about William a lot but knew he was in good hands. I was not in a fit state to make the journey to the hospital to see him so I just rested and waited for news.

The phone call I received that Monday really worried me. Despite being given full-dose broad-spectrum, third generation antibiotics my patient was no better.

I gave Professor Munro a ring.

'He's a mystery, Peter,' said the great man. 'I was sure he had a leak which would be covered by the ileostomy but I could not prove it. I cannot find anything else. I do not think going back into his tummy is the right move. I think we must wait it out.'

'OK, but let me know what goes. I will try and be in on Wednesday.'

By Wednesday I was in a fit enough condition to climb in my car and get to the hospital. Instead of mounting the eight flights of stairs in my usual fitness regime my secretary was surprised to see that I took the lift.

I popped onto the ward to see William before I started my clinic.

The bay where he had been monitored close to the nursing station was empty.

'He was shifted to ICU at about four o'clock this morning,' said a staff nurse as if it was not a particularly interesting or significant a development.

'Christ!' I moaned and went hurtling down the stairs nearly falling in the process as I forgot that I had hardly been able to stand up the day before.

In ICU I found William on a ventilator being given inotropic, or cardiac, drug support.

'It's not looking good, Peter,' said a sympathetic intensivist.

'Have we had any more scans?' I asked weakly.

'Yes we've had a shed load but they have not really told us what the problem is.'

I cannot really express the misery that a complication of this sort after one of my operations gives me. It is a combination of fear, guilt and self-loathing, as I reason that something that I have done has led to the catastrophe I can see unfolding before my eyes. It is like a slow-motion road traffic accident.

Over the years I have experienced this feeling more times than I would like to remember. The guilt of feeling that I have caused harm by an operation I have carried out. The sin of commission rather than the lesser sin of omission, as in mistaking a diagnosis or failing to act. That somehow seems easier to bear. Although both sins are miserable for a doctor and a patient to experience, I know from bitter experience that the sin of commission hurts more.

Often I have had the fantasy, that if I could monetise the problem, and pay money to the Devil, if necessary, to make my patient well again, I would do so.

In cash.

Now.

No questions asked.

To any God or Devil that might help me.

The intensivist soon woke me from my torment.

'No more scans booked today. We think he is too ill to move to get another CT or MRI. We could get the radiologist to come down and run an ultrasound over him,' he said.

'Good idea! Anything to give us a clue. Call me as soon as they're here.'

An hour later I got a call from the radiologist.

'Your patient has had his scan and I think he's got a necrotic gall-bladder. No gall stones but I think he has had acute gangrenous cholecystitis.'

'What? Really? Why now? He never had gall-bladder problems before and it has nothing to do with my operation or his cancer.'

'Yes I understand that but the gall-bladder wall is thickened and looks to me like it has perforated.'

'My God, that explains it all. Nothing to do with my operation. Just a bloody coincidence. I had better get him into theatre as soon.'

The intensivist he shook his head and look worried.

'He's not very good, Peter. Not much reserve. Blood pressure sagging substantially. Is there any other way?'

'I am afraid not.'

'Are you up for it, Peter? You look bloody awful.'

'Yeah I'll be all right but I will ask Professor Munro to come and assist too if he can.'

It was another hour before the patient was in theatre anaesthetised. A ventilated patient already in ICU does not need much anaesthesia as they are half way there already. Just a shot of morphine and some muscle relaxant and we were ready to start.

As I opened the abdomen through my previous incision a rush of bile stained fluid emerged. I noticed also fibrinous adhesions covering the surface of the small bowel. This is normal in late peritonitis and is a worrying sign. It means that the perforation has been in existence for quite a while.

Bile peritonitis, as it is called when the bile leaks from the gall-bladder, is a particularly capricious enemy because the inflammation the bile causes is not very marked at first. Bile, unlike gastric contents from a perforated duodenal ulcer, does not produce much pain initially. Insidiously it acts as a gentle chemical irritant and then, bit by bit, bacterial peritonitis becomes established. Then, before anyone quite realizes, the patient starts to tumble down, what I call, the septic cascade. If they fall too far they will not be able to climb back up even with surgical or medical help. When sepsis like this is left too long the patient cannot recover.

Sure, enough William's inflamed gall-bladder was perforated and leaking bile, a consequence of having lost its blood supply. I had seen this a half dozen times before. Sometimes it is spontaneous and occasionally after another event like a heart attack, a major operation or a concomitant illness. But being a relative rarity, it can catch the doctors out. One of the difficulties is that the CT scan, which is a first-class way of looking deep into body cavities, is not a particularly good method for investigating gall-bladder disease. Ultrasound is a better method.

This had been the case with William.

Damn it! We had all been barking up the wrong tree.

Assisted by Professor Munro, who was as surprised as I had been to learn of the diagnosis, I took out the gall-bladder, sewed up the cystic duct that connects with the common bile duct and washed out the peritoneum and closed the abdomen. The operation was without complication and there was hardly any bleeding. But William was now on maximum cardiac support and oxygen. His blood pressure was dropping.

After a phone call to his wife, I realised I was going to collapse imminently. The emotional strain, the emergency operation and the virus were a lethal cocktail. I was finished. It was all I could do to limp to my car and drive home. The next day I was laid up in bed again. It seemed the exertions of the day before had put my own recovery back some days. I took a couple of paracetamol and a tot of whisky and tried to get some rest.

I got the news about William in the middle of the next night. I went down to the kitchen so as not to disturb Christina.

It was the intensivist on the line.

'I am sorry to tell you, Peter, but William died tonight at midnight despite all our efforts.'

'Oh, Lord! We got there too late,' I groaned. 'My God, what terrible news.'

I paused for a moment thinking how everyone involved must be feeling.

'Sorry to have put you to all that trouble. Goodnight', I said apologetically. I put the phone down and stared out of the kitchen window. Suddenly the night seemed darker and my bronchitic breathing already worsened by the flu became more laboured.

I stared at the wall in front of me without hearing Christina calling down to see if everything was OK.

Without warning standing in the kitchen by the phone that had conveyed this most terrible of news, I found myself weeping uncontrollably.

***

I had written about burn-out and stress before it truly happened to me that night when William died. I had suffered times of stress in relation to my patients but this was the worst it had ever been. Within a few days I was experiencing guilt accompanied by an acute crisis of confidence.

As I suffered, I remembered a surgical friend who had gassed himself in his car. A patient, on whom he had carried out a gastrectomy for stomach cancer, had sustained a fatal complication after his surgery. My friend was a newly appointed consultant in a teaching hospital working alongside a fairly unsympathetic group of surgical colleagues. They did not know him well. In consequence, when the disaster occurred, he had no-one in the hospital to share the burden of guilt with. In addition, he was alone. He had no partner and his much beloved mother had died a month before.

He was a fine, kind and caring surgeon. He had a brilliant future ahead when he had placed that hose in the exhaust pipe and wound up the windows of his Volkswagen Passat in the hospital carpark. He had turned the engine on and had died quickly.

He was just thirty-nine years old.

His death had affected many deeply. I suppose his colleagues had not recognised the danger he was in or they would have stepped in to help. Inadvertently they had let him wallow in the blame that he had piled on himself.

Thinking of my own failure to diagnose William's condition, I now tumbled down the same spiral staircase of self-loathing. I was very miserable. Unlike that dead friend I, at least, had a loving wife, a family, a wonderful secretary and plenty of good colleagues. Professor Munro recognised my plight when he phoned me the day after William had died.

'Don't blame yourself, Peter. It could not be helped. We all got it wrong.'

'But I cannot but keep blaming myself. I just cannot think of anything else.'

'I fully understand. Why not take some time off? We will cover for your patients. We all understand. I think you should get away for a while.'

And that is what I did.

A day or two at home did not seem to be enough to sort it so, despite the wonderful support groups I possessed, I fled into the hills. I drove three hundred miles to the Lake District and sought out my old Himalayan climbing friends.

A few hard days pushing myself up the peaks might solve my problem. It was clear to me now that this would have to be my escape route.

Two days later, I was scrambling up Scafell Pike (978 metres) in a storm. The cold rain was pricking my skin and the wind was chilling me to the core. Paradoxically, I was enjoying the pain enormously. It stopped me thinking dark thoughts. As I began the climb down to the valley below, I knew I was starting the slow journey to renewal and redemption. As we made the hard descent through Hollow Stones, the storm clouds passed. The sunshine on Wast Water below us raised my spirits further.

The autumn evening was drawing to a close and now the light was fading fast. The last stretch descending to Wasdale Head was fearfully hard on the knees but the bitter beer that we drank on arrival at the hotel was the finest I had ever tasted. After some lamb stew and dumplings and a couple of hours warming in front of the open fire with a wee dram, we found our way to our beds.

That night for the first time in ten days I slept soundly.

During the week I spent in Cumbria, I began to mend. I realised that William's death had not been my fault but a series of circumstances I could not have predicted or prevented. Others had failed too and we had all been fooled. A case of looking the wrong way into the tunnel as the train raced towards us from the other direction.

By the time I got back home to Hertfordshire I was ready again to face the surgical music. I knew the emotional exhaustion that had surfaced in the form of suicidal thoughts was, to some extent, caused by my physical illness. Influenza is often followed by depression and, perhaps, that was part of it too.

Doctors like me are taught and teach a great deal about the fears and anxieties that our patients and relatives may display. But we know little about how to defend ourselves when those fears become our own. The analogy of post-traumatic stress syndrome in a war veteran is an appropriate one.

The term 'second victim' was developed to help us understand that, when a disaster occurs to a patient, the surgeon, who has taken the risk on behalf of his patient, may be another victim. This does not detract from the importance of the first victim in any way, but it acknowledges that there may be more than one party to care for in the aftermath of a complication.

***

The next week, I was able to offer my condolences in person to William's widow. I was dreading the meeting but I knew that both of us would gain from it. I was certainly correct in that regard. As has often happened in my medical career, patients have sustained me as much as vice versa. This was a case in point.

'I am sorry we did not recognise in time what was really happening to William. It was a bad time for me to get ill but I left him in good hands with Professor Munro and he was fooled just as I was.'

'I understand, Mr. McDonald, that you all tried your hardest to save him. William could not say a bad word about you. He knew you had his interests at heart at all times. At least we both had our faith to support us.'

We looked for a moment into each other's eyes and I wondered what she was thinking. Indirectly because of what I had attempted to do for her husband to cure his rectal cancer, she was now a widow looking forward to a lonelier retirement than she had anticipated. But, although I knew that I had not caused the cancer or the gallbladder perforation, I could not but feel that I had failed them both.

When commentators talk about surgeons being bold, brash and even callous they completely miss the point. Surgeons and others may have to appear to be so in order to protect themselves from the mistakes that they will inevitably make in the course of their work. Each surgeon will cope with this in their own way. I have a tendency to blame myself. Others like to blame the system. The weakest ones try and blame the patient's pre-existing illnesses or their failure to call for help in time.

Perhaps it would be nice to believe in Fate. I once had a colleague who was such a devout Christian that, when his patients suffered a complication at his hands, he did not blame himself but was happy to put the responsibility clearly where it lay.

With God.

It was surely the Deity who had failed to guide his hands that day. What a lovely insurance policy that must have been for that surgeon.

I have often wished I had that faith and that belief. I think it would made have many aspects of the life I have pursued easier than it has been.

But on the other hand, it might have blunted the highs and lows and resulted in a life with less contrast.

My professional life has certainly not felt like a life of mediocrity. I am not alone thinking this.

Ask any surgeon.

***

This sad tale concluded with an escape to the hills to clear the torment in my soul. It is often said that a change is as good as a rest. Perhaps, that is why so many of us crave vacations in order to recharge the batteries or maybe it is to understand again and again that the grass is not necessarily greener elsewhere.

Chapter 14:
How Overseas Visits Allow Me To Take Stock

❖

In 1983, when I was a middle grade registrar in Southampton, I began to pen a series of articles reporting from other countries for the magazine Hospital Doctor. I had always fancied myself as a foreign correspondent having listened to the BBC all my childhood. I was curious to find out more of how medicine was organised elsewhere.

I had met a young doctor who was a keen flyer and was in possession of a private pilot's licence. Somehow, I managed to persuade the editor of the newspaper to support the expense of renting a light aircraft to get me around northern Europe to interview some foreign doctors. In addition, the editor was generous enough to continue paying my modest fees for the articles and help with accommodation and the fuel expenses of the plane. It was a win/win as my friend wanted to increase his flying hours so he bore the cost of the hiring of the little Cessna aircraft himself. When I look back on that time, my editor must have had a chest full of money that needed spending because I later discovered that editors are notoriously mean with expenses.

Over the course of the next year, we flew together through the clouds to Cork, Guernsey, Lille, Amsterdam, Paris and Ostend from Eastleigh Airport near Southampton. We usually departed on Saturday lunchtime and landed well before dark. I would then walk into the biggest hospital in the city and begin interviewing the first doctors I met. Within an hour or two, I would have enough information to write up my copy before we headed off to the best restaurant we could find to enjoy the local food and wine. On Sunday afternoon, we would head for home ready for work the next day.

I was in a kind of journalist's paradise.

It all went to plan until we tried to take off from Schiphol Airport in Amsterdam one Sunday evening. The plane had a flat battery. Despite all our efforts we were grounded until a new battery could be charged up. It was a blow for I knew I would be late for my professor's breakfast meeting at 7.30am the next morning at the Royal South Hants Hospital. So, I telephoned my colleagues to relay the message to the team. Needless to say, the professor was not impressed but he was generous enough to tolerate my thirst for knowledge if not my tardiness. He was a kindly, quiet sort of man. His integrity and hard work ethos were never in doubt and he had both good clinical judgement and a fine pair of hands.

But he could make no small talk whatsoever.

A week later at the next Monday breakfast session he gave me a wry look as we sat down to croissants and coffee to review the patients for the week.

'Nice to see you are here this Monday morning, Peter,' he began sarcastically.

'Yes, Prof, sorry about the flat battery in the aircraft last week. It seems a poor excuse but it really did happen,' I pleaded hoping he believed me.

'Ah yes, a flat battery? An unlikely story but so original that it must be true?' he joked.

There was an embarrassing silence.

He smiled awkwardly.

From past experience we knew the lull might last many minutes. We were prepared for a long wait. The good professor never seemed to be uncomfortable with the length of these pauses.

We sat patiently but on this occasion, we did not have to wait long.

Suddenly this quietly mannered senior academic looked up to the ceiling and shrieked.

'Aaaaagh!!! Ooooh! Ooooh! Ooooh! Aaaaagh!!!'

Mouths open the whole surgical team watched in awe as the professor jumped up and down like a jack-in-a-box in the breakfast canteen. With the screams piercing through to the wards above, he pulled down his trousers and ran out of the room. There was a scampering noise on the floor as the rat, which had obviously climbed up his trouser leg, made his escape to the kitchens nearby.

It was a scene that would be worthy of any French farce. By the time the professor returned in his boxer shorts to retrieve his trousers, the laughter of the team had only just died down.

After such an escapade the fact that I had been late for the breakfast meeting the week before was completely forgotten.

My bacon had been saved by a rodent.

**

To complement my airborne reportage, I would add to my series of foreign reports when I was away at surgical conferences. In that way, I reported directly from Copenhagen and Athens. I also interviewed visiting doctors from many other countries. By this second-hand method, I published articles on medicine in the Soviet Union, Canada, Brazil, Japan, Switzerland and Sweden. Another time in 1984, when I was on my way to climb Mt. Kenya with a couple of my old mountaineering friends, our Egyptair 707 developed an engine fault. We had purchased cheap tickets so we were grounded for a week in Cairo. I took this unexpected opportunity to interview Dr. Haney Sami, a senior house officer, at the Qasr-el-Aini hospital, which dates back to the seventh century AD.

Another scoop in the bag!

It was exhilarating being a roving international reporter. I imagined that I was a Times foreign correspondent and that millions were reading my reports. Although the readership of Hospital Doctor was calculated at 40,000 souls, in reality, I expect many threw this free magazine out with the rubbish unread. It is man's folly to dream dreams but, at least, in 1986 I put the experience to good use when working at the Cleveland Clinic, Ohio by sending back weekly pieces on the state of US medicine. There my fantasy took another turn as I pictured myself as the medical equivalent of one of my journalist heroes, Alastair Cooke.

I took this even further when I persuaded the Queensland Broadcasting Company to use me as their UK radio correspondent. The time difference meant that I could speak live at 11pm before heading to bed. Unfortunately, they soon realised I knew nothing of football and even less about minor celebrities so dumped me after only six months.

On my visits to these hospitals in so many countries, I observed there was much wasted medical manpower. Many young doctors would be trained but not all would practise medicine. Where there is not a fixed numerus clausus, or quota system, as there is in Britain with its limited number of medical student places, the wastage is greatest. In France this amounted to 70 per cent of medical students failing to qualify while in Denmark, where the reduction in the hours of work had created many new junior posts, thousands were treading water as all the senior permanent posts above them were already filled.

My reports took many forms and once when this budding colorectal surgeon was sailing one summer in the Aegean Sea on a boat misappropriately named Ainos, he found himself on the Greek island of Sciathos. Noting its 5,000 inhabitants I headed for the local hospital and clinic. The island had three doctors who were general practitioners in the old sense.

The hospital, or nosokomio, was opposite the church and the best taverna. It was tiny. Clinics and emergency treatments were carried out locally while seriously ill patients were transferred to Athens by helicopter. There was an air of sleepiness in the Greek health system both in Sciathos and, when I went later to a huge city hospital in Athens, I found it was the same there. Perhaps it mirrored the heat of the day and the phlegmatism of the people.

The poorly paid doctor I interviewed about the Soviet Union and its hospitals had worked for a time for an ambulance service with a couple of nurses. He had noted that the best paid crew member was actually the driver of the vehicle not the medics. The method of achieving promotion in the USSR was by joining the Communist Party. It seemed that the whole megalithic medical machine was extraordinarily inefficient grinding along with a magnificent slowness almost to the point of paralysis.

The long-standing joke about the efficiency of Marxism might apply also to the way medicine was run in that country:

Question: 'What will life be like in the Sahara when socialism comes to that region?'

Answer: 'They will run out of sand.'

History in the end proved that it was socialism that ran out before the sand but, as I have worked in and observed the British NHS for more than fifty years, I wonder if we are not simulating the same centralised, top-down model of care with its gross inefficiencies.

In all the countries I reported, the doctors were still at the top of the list of professions trusted by the public. Even the low salaries offered in the Soviet Union had not reduced the respect doctors were given, much in the same way as the nineteenth century local government 'zemstvo' doctors, who laboured in the isolated towns and villages of rural Russia on very low stipends, were thought of a century and a half ago.

In Canada the specialists largely worked without junior doctors supporting them so the pyramid of progression was flatter. There was therefore no need to languish year after year in training posts as we were forced to do in Britain.

Surely if any country could get it right it would be the Swiss? Not entirely, I discovered. The frustrations of the doctors were palpable there. The power of the head of department médecin chef or chef artz was absolute and the system very vertically hierarchical compared with the horizontally orientated we-are-all equal consultant system in the UK.

A horizontal system with equal teams treating their own patients independently, at least, means that a rogue head of department can be neutralised easily. Sometimes this is not the case within the continental medical command structures where a bad chief can destroy a service entirely before he can be stopped. With first, second and third class patients being treated all differently, the Swiss were not so concerned about equality but, at least, none of their patients had to wait long for their treatments. Very different from the UK where months and even years of waiting is possible.

In Egypt, my attention was held not by the medical aspects of the hospital but by its lack of nurses. There was hardly a nurse in sight. Relatives were sleeping by the side of their loved ones' beds attending to their needs. Although 85% of medical students in Egypt will qualify, the shortage of jobs and the poor wages means that many go to the UAE, United States or Saudi Arabia to work. With tuberculosis, bilharzia, polio and rheumatic fever, the doctors who stayed in Cairo had their work cut out.

In highly populated Brazil there were plenty of doctors but, after discussing their country with three visiting Brazilian surgeons, I had the distinct impression that many citizens were left out of the system as were some of the doctors. There were many unemployed or under-employed doctors. Some had to supplement their incomes by working outside medicine driving taxis or doing other casual work. However, the pace of medicine was different for those in work. The Brazilian surgeons I interviewed had seen me work in the British NHS and were unimpressed.

'At home I never have to plough through a clinic of forty people in an afternoon like you do,' said one.

'How old are you?' they asked.'

'Thirty-four,' I replied.

'Thirty-four and still not a consultant? In Brazil that would be inconceivable.'

Despite the trio of homesick Brazilian surgeons, or cirurgiãos extolling the wonderful land they lived in, I had a feeling that the real and massive problems of health provision in their country were being largely ignored. Poverty, malnutrition, intestinal parasites and high child mortality. Mainly these surgeons seemed to be doctors keen to treat the middle and upper classes only.

Although many are forced to wait a long time in England for a consultant post, it was worse in Japan. As my editor had refused point blank to fly me to Tokyo, I commissioned a friend to interview a surgeon in Nagao City University Hospital. Seventeen years after qualifying as a doctor this surgeon still had not reached independent practice status. In Japan healthcare is divided 50:50 between public and private, and there is no medical unemployment. Without a developed primary healthcare system, medical treatment is largely hospital based, so was more expensive for the state.

What did my readers and I learn from these medical fishing expeditions? We learnt that pursuing a medical career was competitive everywhere but conditions of work and prospects for promotion were very different in each country. At least, in all countries doctors were respected and nearly all were paid adequately.

There were plenty of variations in all jurisdictions with the administrative systems that had been developed to deliver healthcare.

It certainly was not a case of one-size-fits-all.

***

There are few professional qualifications recognised in every country in the world. Medicine, nursing and its allied professions are probably the most transferable skills on the planet. All other disciplines are parochial. Law, business, journalism, and politics are all very dependent on where they are practised.

By the beginning of the twentieth century when scientific methodology led to extraordinary discoveries, medicine in its present allopathic form became both universally desirable and the international norm.

My thoughts on this subject are not original. William Osler (1849-1920), a renowned physician, stated more than a hundred years ago that:

'Medicine is the only worldwide profession, following everywhere the same methods, actuated by the same ambitions and pursuing the same ends.'

I suppose modern aviation might be similar. Airline pilots can work almost anywhere, but that is a very small group of individuals flying planes around the world that are essentially identical. A minor activity compared with medicine.

To illustrate my argument, I can boast that I have given the same lecture in Peru one week and India the next. In both places the interest was the same, the discussions equally sophisticated and the debates well-informed. Without trying too hard on the international circuit during my medical career, I have been fortunate to work in seven countries and given lectures in twenty-eight. These overseas visits are important. They both break up the monotony of routine and also provide important cross-fertilisation of ideas.

***

One such memorable visit was when I went as a visiting professor to the Lebanese Society for General Surgery in June 2013. The year before that visit I had been President of the Section of Surgery at the Royal Society of Medicine and I had been approached by a Lebanese professor of surgery to take a delegation to his homeland.

I had little knowledge of his country and most of what I knew was unfavourable. It had suffered greatly through recent civil war but now was trying to climb out of its misery and join the world again. Hence the invitation. Indeed, the British government was actively encouraging visits to the Lebanon at the time.

I knew that in the 1960s the country had been called 'the Switzerland of the East'. It was said to have been a paradise then. You could swim in the Mediterranean from a quiet beach in the morning and then be skiing on Mount Lebanon in the afternoon. But, as if to bring that idyll into focus, this little country is surrounded by Israel and Syria - an unhappy pair of neighbours.

With its diverse population of 54% Muslims and 40% Christians and many other sub-tribes including Druse, it was governed by an unstable alliance. I was aware that the terrible civil war between 1975 and 1990 had practically destroyed the country's infrastructure but that this was now over. The Lebanon was trying hard to rebuild.

Although some of my surgical colleagues in London refused my offer to travel to an area of potential strife, I was able to recruit five others to come with me. In early June 2013, we found ourselves flying out of London on a nearly empty Middle East Airlines Airbus

A330 to the Eastern Mediterranean. As we cruised in clear skies at 38,000ft above Cyprus I could see that troubled island laid out before me. This region, once known as the Levant, has always been a cauldron and there is not a country in the region without the scars of recent war. All had continuing major political problems.

The Mediterranean, this beautiful, calm protected sea, and the territories surrounding it, has been fought over since ancient times. Trade by sea and land has been well established over millennia. The climate is warm, the land fertile and the people resourceful. Phoenicians, Carthaginians, Eqyptians, Greeks, Roman, Normans, Moors, Ottomans, Barbary pirates, Frenchmen and Britons. All had made their mark by offering trade, often with the threat of violence.

The Phoenicians, who had originated from the Levant, had spread throughout the Mediterranean. They were adept merchants, expert seafarers, and intrepid explorers. Their modern counterparts from the Lebanon are not dissimilar with their highly successful diaspora all over the world but particularly in South America. These migrants send large quantities of money back home. Despite its political problems the Lebanon can still boast that it has one of the highest per capita income countries in the Middle East.

I remember the view as we approached Beirut from the west just before sunset. I was surprised just how dramatic its setting was. High-rise buildings casting long shadows as far as I could see. These tower blocks were stacked together on the coastline peninsula that is Beirut as well as high up on the foothills of the Mount Lebanon range of mountains. I could see the high point of the mountain at 3,500 metres in the distance as the aircraft glided down towards the city.

My first impression was this looked much like Rio de Janeiro. Mountains sweeping down to the sea sheltering a huge city on their lower slopes behind a coastal corniche. The plane landed and we made our way to the Hilton Habtool Hotel where our hosts had placed me on the twenty-eighth floor with a view over the city. The staff made sure we were welcomed warmly.

But the news that week had been worrying.

Hezbollah, urged on by Iran, had started fighting the Free Syrian Army on the northern borders of the Lebanon, while other Sunni groups were taking pot shots at the Shias in the suburbs of Tripoli, the Lebanon's second largest city. The Lebanese army, comprising a weak coalition of Christians, Druse, and Muslims, were trying to referee the fighting but it only seemed a matter of time before it would spread to the outskirts of Beirut. This recent disturbance would be the vindication for some of my colleagues. When I had invited them to join me, they had decided to stay safe at home taking heed of a recent warning from the UK's Foreign and Commonwealth Office to avoid venturing into this land of multiple religious and ethnic groups all pulling in different directions.

Later that evening we were taken to a fine restaurant where a mezze of Lebanese traditional dishes and wines were waiting for us. I knew that the food in Lebanon would be good. It consists of an abundance of whole grains, fruits, vegetables, fresh fish and seafood. Poultry is eaten more often than red meat, which is usually lamb and goat. Garlic and olive oil, often seasoned with lemon juice, is used in large quantity and the dishes of falafel, shawarma, hummus, tabbouleh, and sesame tahini complement any savoury meal.

Always one to oblige my generous hosts, I forced down a mouthful of raw liver, sowda, but tried not to think of the parasites that might be lurking within. Baklava and meghli for dessert were washed down with some arak, an anise liqueur, the Lebanese national drink but, after declining more, I soon found myself with a glass of extraordinarily good red wine.

I had believed wrongly that it must have been the short French colonisation of Lebanon (1923-1946) that had brought wine to the area but that was not the case. Although the French Mandate in the Lebanon encouraged wine production, the Lebanon is among the oldest sites of wine production in the world. Indeed, the Israelite prophet Hosea (780–725 BC) urged his followers to return to God so that: 'They will blossom as the vine and fame be like the wine of Lebanon.'

The Phoenicians spread wine and viticulture throughout the Mediterranean and, despite the unrest in the country, the Lebanon still has an annual production of more than eight million bottles with the centre of that production being in the wide, fertile Bekaa Valley to the East of Mount Lebanon.

That night I slept well and early the next morning the conference began. Our hosts were effusive in their praise of my little delegation, commending us for having made the journey despite the ever-present dangers that the Lebanon is exposed to. Repaying the hospitality, the British surgeons made every effort to deliver first-class lectures to this highly educated, multi-lingual audience from all around the Middle East. Until then I had not appreciated that English in Beirut was only the third language after Arabic and French.

It was a packed hall and our lectures were well received. The audience was a mix of trainee surgeons and established consultants. In the questions and answers sessions I noticed how the older professors, many well over seventy, would pontificate on a matter not offering much scientific reasoning behind their opinions. I imagined that much of the teaching of medicine and surgery in the Lebanon was didactic and accompanied by little debate.

Notwithstanding this, the debates on the presentations we had brought with us – *Operative Treatment of Abdominal Sarcoma, Laparoscopic Rectal Cancer Excision* and *Acute Cholecystitis* – were vigorous and interesting. By 6pm we were ready to get back to the hotel for a swim before we were driven to the British Ambassador's residence. Although the food served was not of the quality of the feast the night before, Ambassador Tom Fletcher was warm in his welcome. It was clear he was a great friend of the country.

While in Beirut, Fletcher had pioneered a more open style of diplomacy and the BBC had even made a documentary about him titled *The Naked Diplomat*. He had led UK initiatives on refugee education, job creation and border security. *The Daily Telegraph* reported that he was behind a secret plan to prevent Islamic State from entering the Lebanon from Syria. Indeed, the UK government's aid budget for the Lebanon had increased from £2m in 2011 to £200m in 2015 by the time Fletcher had stepped down from his post. Although I am not a professional ambassador-watcher, this seems to have been no mean achievement for a diplomat in a short span of time.

As the week wore on I was more and more impressed by the resourceful Lebanese and their worldly, cosmopolitan and business-orientated outlook. In Beirut it seemed that there was enterprise, energy and hospitality on a grand scale. Somewhat to my surprise, there was also great wealth and corruption sitting side by side with significant poverty. Not a recipe for a peaceful society in the long term.

On the last day of the visit we were driven to Byblos, modern Jbail, where the first alphabet had been invented by those clever Phoenicians. The Bible derives its title from this settlement's name, which means *papyrus*.

In a seashore restaurant a lunch hosted by the Minister of Tourism, a man who had the rare talent of being able to gobble up his tabbouleh while simultaneously conducting a TV interview extolling the importance our visit. A quick swim from off the stern of a speedboat and back to Beirut for the final day of conference. I joked that we should point the boat south at 40 knots and see how far we could get.

'Just two hours later you would be entering Israeli waters and either be in the hands of the Israeli Defence Force or blown out of the water by a Typhoon 30mm cannon fired from a Super Dvora Mk III,' said my host not exaggerating.

I stopped making bad jokes after that sobering thought.

A final gala dinner that evening completed our extraordinary visit to this little Middle Eastern country. There was much triple-kissing, hand-shaking and even some dancing to seal our new-found friendships. I flew home next day thinking that the Lebanon's problems were lessening and that a bright future might be dawning.

Wishful thinking. Wrong again.

Since then refugees from Syria have continued to pour in, putting impossible strains on the country. In 2020, Beirut experienced both Covid-19 and a catastrophic inadvertent bomb blast that wiped out a quarter of the city. Demonstrations and clashes recently reflect significant growing tensions between Christian and Muslim groups. In just a few months the political class has been discredited and all the leaders replaced.

It seems likely that the Lebanon will be not be a tranquil place in the years to come. But it will still be populated by some of those sophisticated, generous people that I met during that visit back in 2013.

With such time spent overseas, it can truly be said that medicine certainly reaches the parts that other professions cannot. But now I must return again to the United Kingdom where a two decades earlier migration of a tiny hospital altered my professional life forever.

Chapter 15:
St. Mark's Hospital Comes To Harrow

❖

I cannot remember exactly when my gastroenterology colleague, Jonathan Levi, sat me down in his office. Maybe it was autumn 1992 or just after.

'Peter, what would you say to St. Mark's Hospital relocating to Harrow and joining us at Northwick Park?'

'Er? Merging with us? Coming over here lock stock and barrel?'

'Yes. They need to be near a big hospital for theatres, intensive care and other services. St. Bartholomew's Hospital is the obvious place for them to team up with but they have failed to agree. Something about loss of identity by being swallowed by the bigger hospital. So they want to come here. What do you think?'

It took me only a couple of minutes to weigh up the pros and cons.

I knew St. Mark's well. I had been clinical fellow there in the early eighties and had even published a seminal paper with one of the St. Mark's surgeons on the most unglamorous topic of anal fissure. A few years later in 1989 I had been a resident surgical officer (RSO) on secondment from Southampton where I was a lecturer in surgery. I recalled the hard graft working at St. Mark's. Being the only doctor at night and weekends in the little hospital with sixty beds had been tough. It was both lonely and scary and when a patient got critically ill, I would have to ship them out to St. Bartholomew's for intensive care.

I had travelled up on the train each Monday morning at the crack of dawn from Southampton and cycled across Waterloo Bridge. I would pick my way through Holborn and Clerkenwell to reach the hospital on City Road.

St. Mark's was founded in 1835 by Frederick Salmon, a surgeon who could not get a post at St. Bartholomew's Hospital. Being an outsider to London from the city of Bath, he had been turned down for promotion on no less than four occasions. With others he had exposed and spoken out about the corruption of how appointments to hospitals were made. Patronage and nepotism, not merit, was the prevailing ethos and the newly formed Lancet medical journal was campaigning hard for change.

Pointing out the deficiencies in the system Salmon, like me one-hundred and seventy years later, was black-balled. He eventually decided to bypass this mire of patronage and with the help of some City of London businessmen founded his Infirmary for the Relief of the Poor Afflicted with Fistula and Other Diseases of the Rectum. He felt passionately that this area of medicine had been neglected by the big hospitals and that he might make a contribution by specialising in it. It was the first hospital in the world to focus on this unfashionable region of the body. New York's Proctology Hospital followed more than sixty years later in 1895.

St. Mark's became a busy place quite quickly and even Charles Dickens had been treated there for an anal fistula in 1841. The novelist and campaigner expressed 'a spontaneous and heartfelt emotion of gratitude' to Salmon. The operation to eradicate this chronic infection around his anus was followed by a modest donation of £10 (£1,040 in today's money) from Dickens, who was then appointed a governor.

After two moves this tiny hospital relocated to the City Road, Islington in 1853 and perhaps became the only hospital in the world with 'etc.' in its title as St. Mark's Hospital for Fistula etc. was inscribed in stone on its facade. In an odd way this awkward title earned the hospital a certain notoriety although it continued to juggle with many name changes over the next hundred years.

***

My time at St. Mark's Hospital had been fruitful. Being an RSO was a sort of rite de passage with its hardships and long hours. To be a card-carrying colorectal surgeon in the UK, St. Mark's was as good a ticket as any to have. Indeed, when I have lectured to surgeons around the globe they have all known of the famous St. Mark's Hospital but none have been able to say what the oldest hospital in England, St. Bartholomew's Hospital, was noted for.

So, this was the institution wanting to join us at Northwick Park?

It would mean merging services but preserving the identity of the two hospitals to keep both brands intact. There would be more competition for the work between the greater number of consultants but a bigger pool of expertise which would bring with it many new opportunities for teaching and research. All these thoughts went through my head. My answer was unequivocal.

'Great idea Jonathan. When can they start?'

Thus began a year of meetings and much planning.

Firstly between the clinicians and then involving the administrators and finally the politicians.

I was appointed as a consultant at St. Mark's the following year and began to work in City Road one day a week. It all went to plan and in the summer of 1995, St. Mark's moved on to the Northwick Park Hospital site. There was plenty of space as a large part of the hospital had become vacant because the Medical Research Council, who had run out of money, had decided to close their custom-made Clinical Research Centre on the site.

St. Mark's Hospital could now concentrate on growing its services. It had been the world leader in many aspects of colorectal diseases but there were now many other centres in the UK that had strong reputations for teaching and research in the same field. Although pioneering work on cancer, ulcerative colitis and Crohn's Disease, incontinence, fistulas and polyposis had been the hallmark of St. Mark's, other institutions were steaming ahead with minimally invasive treatments and robotic rectal cancer surgery.

As I reflect today on the last twenty-five years since that move took place, by any measure St. Mark's has done well in its new location. More consultants, more patients, more research and more teaching than ever before. But the strains of sharing a site with a huge, busy general hospital with the pressure of its emergency patients has slowly whittled down St. Mark's' ability to get some of its national referral work done. With Covid-19 in recent months these strains have become even more acute as non-Covid-19 elective or even semi-urgent operations have no so-called 'clean site' to be admitted to.

Hospitals are not static organisations. They must adapt or die just as St. Mark's, which had begun as Salmon's Infirmary in 1835, had metamorphosed, shifting its footprint three times before ending up in Harrow. It seems today that another move to an intermediate site is now probable. St. Mark's was situated on City Road for one hundred and forty-two years but only twenty-six years after arriving on the Northwick Park site, it could be on the move again.

I wonder how long it will survive in its next incarnation.

***

Men and women go to work for a number of reasons. To earn a living, to socialise, to gain self-esteem through status which comes from achievement or simply to have a routine with the discipline that accompanies it. A hospital fulfils all these needs when morale is high. Despite the responsibilities inherent in the job of treating patients, if a hospital is in fine form every stress is bearable.

St. Mark's is small enough to feel like a family. With probably only two hundred active employees everyone knows everyone. One barometer of morale is the hospital's Christmas pantomime, when the junior staff mock the consultants mercilessly and the consultants retaliate with a sketch or two in return. If the workers can laugh together they will work better together to care for those that are dying or in distress.

Even more important is the comfort they can give each other in the hard tasks they must perform. Team work is nowadays the buzz phrase. Sometimes it is self-evident that team work is vital to any undertaking while at other times articulating it almost sounds like an irrelevant cliché.

I will illustrate the importance of teamwork by citing the case of Gordon.

**

Gordon came to see me in my private clinic at St. Mark's one Wednesday afternoon. I knew him well as I had removed his anus and rectum for cancer fifteen years previously. He had been about fifty then. His tumour had responded well to pre-operative chemotherapy and radiotherapy so that, when I removed it six months later, there was only a small residual of cancer left. Better still, the lymph nodes draining the rectum were free from cancer. This gave him a good prognosis and this had turned out to be the case.

Now at nearly sixty-five he was in good health apart from having put on a few more kilograms than his wife would have liked. Recurrence at this late stage would be most unusual so I had long since considered him cured.

His colostomy, which he managed by irrigating every morning, had not misbehaved much over the years even though it is known that the longer a patient has a colostomy the more likely it is to cause problems. It can either prolapse or retract, or more commonly develop a hernia of the abdominal wall next to it. This may make keeping a bag on the stoma difficult. It can also become intermittently painful when the small intestine gets stuck, or 'incarcerated', within the hernia. I have had to repair plenty of these stomal hernias over the years, often with sutures or I sometimes use a piece of mesh.

That morning Gordon was cheerful but a bit fed up with things.

'Mr. McDonald, I keep getting these episodes of pain. The bulge next to the stoma gets tense and the colostomy stops working for a while. After a few hours it settles down but last month I had to be admitted to Watford Hospital for three days and be put on a drip. They did a CT scan and said it was the hernia causing the trouble. Is it time for you to fix it as you threatened a couple of years ago?'

I had seen Gordon every three years for colonoscopy ever since his cancer operation to make sure he had no more polyps appearing in the remaining colon. He had mentioned the problem with the stoma and the accompanying pains before. I had judged that the laterally placed stomal hernia was the cause of his ills and one day a local repair to reduce the hernia and tighten the abdominal wall might be in his interest.

'Well, Gordon I think you are right. Time to fix it. Should take an hour but no more and I will keep you in for a couple of nights at the most. If we use your insurance policy we could get that sorted in the next month.'

So it was that Gordon was admitted to the private ward at St. Mark's three weeks later. He was duly put to sleep and I prepped his abdomen after removing the colostomy bag. I could appreciate the hernia as a definite bulge even though he was lying flat and asleep on the operating table. Of course, when he had been standing up in the clinic it was much more prominent.

I made an L-shaped incision below and to the side of the stoma. Trying desperately to avoid contamination from stool, I dissected out the hernial sac consisting of the peritoneum and excised it. I divided any adhesions attached to the muscle. These fibrous bands can form at any time after the trephine, or hole, is fashioned to bring out the end of the colon. It was quite a deep, narrow cavity due to Gordon's weight gain and it was difficult to expose the area I needed to see. I judged a couple of well-placed sturdy nylon sutures would approximate the muscle and keep the aperture small.

It is a fine judgement to know exactly how small to make the trephine in the abdominal wall when the sutures are finally tied. Too tight and I risked Gordon's colon becoming obstructed again while too lax and the hernia would, as likely as not, return quite quickly.

I tied the two deep full-thickness nylon sutures one after another, leaving just enough room to get the tips of my index and middle finger through the gap remaining alongside the colon.

I judged it was snug but not too tight.

No contamination from stool either.

A shot of antibiotic and Bob's your uncle!

Gordon should be home in a day or two if he was lucky.

I was pleased with my afternoon's work.

I drove home content.

When I saw him at noon the next day he was not a happy man. He had started vomiting at 6am and the colostomy had not worked at all. His abdomen was markedly distended and he was in a moderate degree of pain.

'I don't like the look of this. I think I have tied you up too tight, Gordon. Let me get an X-ray to see if there is any sign this might resolve without me having to take you back to theatre.'

Within an hour I had Gordon's plain abdominal X-ray up on the computer screen at the ward station. It showed gross dilatation of the small bowel and to a lesser extent the large bowel. I must have made the trephine in the abdominal wall too narrow? Surely, there could not be another problem as the obstruction had occurred immediately after my stoma revision. Coincidences like that in medicine can occur but logic told me otherwise in Gordon's case.

'I'll take you back this evening and release the sutures Gordon,' I said.

'But won't the hernia come back and cause me trouble again?'

'I hope not but I cannot be sure. What is clear is I must get you out of obstruction. That must be our first priority. Sorry Gordon.'

A couple of hours later Gordon was in theatre again with a nasogastric tube shoved through his left nostril and down his gullet to drain his stomach. As I scrubbed up for the second time I noticed the content in the gastric bag was very dark green. It signified that the bile that had refluxed back into the stomach from the duodenum where it flows into from the liver was old. This vindicated my decision to take him back to theatre. It meant that the obstruction was severe and likely to be complete and irremediable without surgery.

I reopened the wound next to Gordon's stoma that I had made less than twenty-four hours before. The skin sutures came out easily and the tissue planes were easily prized apart. I could feel the sharp ends of my two nylon sutures and I took the innermost one out first. I decided that both would have to be removed because I could not risk that Gordon would remain obstructed.

The hernia would just have to take its chances. If it recurred I would have to come back and fight another day. The procedure took less than twenty minutes and I felt relieved it was over.

'Thanks Neville,' I said to my anaesthetist, 'fill him up with lots of saline and he should be fine by tomorrow. What a business. Maybe time to give up and find a less stressful job?'

I was sure that Gordon would be fine by the morning.

But Gordon was not fine.

He was still obstructed. Still in pain.

Still producing a huge gastric aspirate.

I could hardly believe my eyes as I examined him. Sometimes guts just go on strike for a few days because they have been interfered with. Surgeons have never quite understood the mechanism of this phenomenon, but was this what was happening here?

'Just got to be patient Gordon. Now I have taken out the sutures it will all get going. Nothing to stop it working now. Just a bit more time.'

I did not sleep well that night. I was mulling it all over in my mind. The condition of bowel obstruction is less dangerous than having peritonitis from a perforated organ with the danger of overwhelming infection, but obstruction of the intestines cannot be sustained for more than a few days. The phrase beloved of old surgeons when they teach their protegés always strikes the fear of God into them.

'Never let the sun rise and fall over a patient with small bowel obstruction!'

In other words, sort out the obstruction before it is too late to save the patient.

Nightmares of Gordon perforating his colon from the build-up of pressure, or getting electrolyte and fluid depleted, swirled around my brain in the early hours. My wife Christina sensed I was not sleeping and asked what the matter was.

'I am really worried about that patient Gordon I told you about. I will have to get someone to come and help me in the morning and give me a second opinion if he is still stuck.'

'Good idea, darling, wise move!' Christina burbled and promptly drifted back to sleep, leaving me alone with my tormented thoughts.

***

It is precisely at times like this that the corporate feeling of working in a well-functioning hospital becomes so important. Northwick Park and now with St. Mark's is full of colleagues who will lend a hand when the need arises. There are some unhelpful colleagues about but they mostly drift off into management jobs or move to some other parts of the health system.

Of course, there's also plenty of competition in the air. Rivalry for influence, position, salary and fame is normal in any organisation and has an important place in keeping up high standards. But there is no deep and sustained personal animosity between any of my colleagues that I know of.

The next morning I saw again that Gordon was no better. He was still obstructed and his stoma bag was completely empty.

'I am going to get an urgent CT scan, Gordon, and get one of my colleagues up to see you before lunchtime and give me a second opinion.'

'Thanks Mr. McDonald. I am sure you will sort me out one way or another. But I do feel very tired and weak.'

Actually, so did I.

My lack of sleep and the strain of the last three days were taking their toll. Worse than that was the fear that I was causing Gordon real harm and might not be able to turn things around. After fixing up the scan and teeing up a theatre for later I phoned a trusted colleague. After explaining the background of Gordon's case I added.

'I think he might have a second problem inside his abdomen such as a tumour or an adhesion but it would be quite a coincidence. I plan to operate on him at about four o'clock if the CT does not suggest anything else. Would you be so kind to come along and assist?'

'Of course, Peter. See you at four. Only too happy to help you out as you have done the same for me on a couple of occasions. Remember that case of biliary peritonitis last year?'

I humoured him as he related the story that he had told me several times before. Strangely, hearing of his previous near disaster took my mind off my own woes for a moment.

Reassured that he would be with me when I operated on Gordon for the third time, I could only wait. The CT scan was equivocal as it so often can be. The radiologist tried to help.

'There is nothing to suggest an unexpected tumour on these scans, Peter. The small bowel is very dilated and there might be a transition point deep in the pelvis but I cannot be certain. Could be a band adhesion but not sure? Doesn't look like it's just a stomal blockage. But some gas is definitely getting through into the stoma bag though I think the obstruction is upstream.'

'Thanks, John. We'll know soon anyway,' I concurred.

I was too polite to suggest that he might be sitting on the fence.

***

I decided to perform a full-blown laparotomy on Gordon by making a moderate sized mid-line incision. It would be more painful afterwards but it would give me enough room to find out what was really happening. If I just went through the twice used L- shaped incision again, I might not be able to see enough. Charles Mayo, a famous surgeon a hundred years ago in America, had advised that all surgeons should expose well and leave a dry field at the end of the operation. I was going to heed his advice on this occasion. Without being dramatic, although Gordon was still holding up, this third operation was rapidly turning into, to use a Yankee expression, the last chance saloon for him.

As well as my colleague Stuart, who had just arrived, Neville, my anaesthetist, was back again in theatre with me. Having both colleagues with me was very reassuring. Although professional pilots now fly unacquainted with their crew members, for surgeons at times of stress a familiar team is very important.

I began my incision, which quickly revealed the grossly distended small bowel. As I opened the abdomen the guts bulged out like those long thin balloons with which you sculpt animals at children's parties.

The ileum, or last part of the small intestine, is only about two centimetres in diameter when empty but Gordon's was ten centimetres across. Muscle thickening, caused by the bowels' peristalsis actions with its attempts to push the contents downstream, added to the distention. The tension in the intestine was so great that at any moment a perforation might occur and liquid stool spill everywhere with dreadful consequences.

I pulled out as much of the small bowel as would come out and wrapped it in warm saline soaked towels to protect it. Deeper inside I discovered a small length of non-dilated small bowel. Between the two was the culprit. A thick band adhesion was straddled tight across the ileum causing near total obstruction. It was far down in the pelvis, thirty centimetres upstream from where my hernia repair had been.

The band must have been there for years waiting for its chance to cause mayhem. It could be a congenital band Gordon had been born with or a post-operative consequence from a previous procedure. All the pains he had experienced running up to his admission at Watford and at St. Mark's were probably due to this band. It really had been an unfortunate coincidence. Damnit! My repair of his hernia had pushed him into complete obstruction.

'Well, my friend, you b******!' I shouted at the band angrily, I think we know what to do with you now!'

Furiously, I divided the band between ligatures as if it was a sentient being. It was thick enough to bleed significantly if I had just sliced through it so I tied the knots carefully. The trapped intestine began to recover immediately. Luckily all of the small bowel was viable. None of it would need to be removed. This would reduce Gordon's chances of having an infection or a leak from a join-up.

As I was feeling confident that now I had found the root cause of his problems, I replaced the two sutures in the muscle to tighten the stoma again. Just enough to repair the hernial defect? Not too tight. It was a small risk but I would not want him to have to go through another procedure to fix his hernia again after this ordeal.

As I placed the full thickness continuous stitch in his abdominal incision I felt happy for the first time in three days. A surgeon's life is full both of misery and wild exhilaration. This had been one of those weeks.

'Thanks for coming along to help me, Stuart. You have been a great moral support.'

Neville, my anaesthetist, who was now getting bored at the top end, began to rib me about this and that. That was a sure sign that he was relaxing too after a few hard hours. More importantly I now considered Gordon out of any real danger. It would take him a few days to get home but he should recover without difficulty now.

And so he did.

Although he had a bit of an ache from his incision and did not get home for a week, he had no more severe pain and no more episodes of obstruction. To my great delight his hernia did not recur, which meant he would not need any further procedure.

Four weeks later I got a note from him and his wife along with four bottles of the finest Scottish malt whisky.

'Yet again Mr. McDonald you pulled out all the stops for me and it has paid off. Thanks a lot and enjoy the fire water!'

Gordon & Naomi

Much to the dismay of Christina, who tries to moderate my taste for whisky, I did indeed enjoy the fire water greatly.

It is always said that whisky tastes better after a long day at work. As I had plenty of long days planned that month, the whisky tasted very fine indeed.

***

St. Mark's Hospital and all the highly motivated staff who work within its walls have come a long way since the hospital's founder decided to start his own infirmary because he could not secure a job at St. Bartholomew's Hospital. A case of success coming from adversity if ever there was.

Many hundreds of thousands of patients over nearly two centuries will be grateful for the failure of Salmon to get preferment. He went on to pioneer an important branch of surgery which had been overlooked until that time. The work of that little hospital with 'etc.' in its title has influenced surgeons all over the world.

After all it must be remembered that there is a Chinese proverb which states:

'Nine out of ten men have piles!'

Coloproctology, as it is now clumsily called, may not seem to be the most glamorous of disciplines.

But it caters for nearly all of us at some time in our lives. It is likely that one day you, the reader, will be in dire need of it.

So best make sure there is a disciple of Frederick Salmon practising somewhere near you.

**

The move of St. Mark's Hospital to Harrow could be said to be a case where management and politics aligned with clinical commonsense. But unfortunately this is not always the case…

Chapter 16:
Why Medical Politicians Sing Out Of Tune

❖

As a young surgeon I was well trained in vascular surgery. I performed many elective and emergency operations on arteries including many aortic aneurysms when the biggest artery in the body starts to leak. When I arrived at Northwick Park Hospital these emergencies were still being carried out by all the general surgeons even if their ordinary daily work was, as in my case, in quite a different field.

I remember in those first couple of years as a consultant I operated on ten emergency leaking aortic aneurysms. These were patients who would inevitably die within a couple of hours if this huge vessel was not replaced by a graft. Oddly my first five patients survived and many thought that I must be an unusually gifted surgeon. Unfortunately the next five patients died, resulting in a mortality rate of 50%, which is about average for that condition in an urban environment where the patients get to hospital quickly. A run of good and then bad luck is not unusual. If the bad run had preceded the good run, questions as to my competency might have been asked. Such runs illustrate the dangers of statistics. Managers should be wary of the perils in store for those that love data more than commonsense.

But I never felt quite at ease with this vascular surgery. Too much blood for my liking. Blood is not really meant to be confined by nylon sutures and Dacron grafts. It can be difficult, scary and frustrating work. When I was a senior registrar I recall assisting an experienced consultant vascular surgeon doing two such aneurysm cases one morning. They took about two hours per case. Unfortunately we were forced to bring them both back to theatre in the afternoon, one after another, for continued bleeding. That was not the end of it because the first one came back to theatre again the same evening.

What a mug's game! Finally when it was possible I was glad to give it all up. The march of sub-specialisation in surgery over the subsequent years has allowed me to pass on this work to our specialist vascular teams, but they too have their moments.

I remember one morning recently, while I was operating on a hot gall-bladder in theatre, our intrepid vascular colleagues were struggling with one such emergency aneurysm in the vascular theatre next door.

The patient, who had been well when he went to bed the night before, was woken with back pain that had got progressively worse. He had noticed that his abdomen was swollen and when he got out of bed he had fainted. His wife had called for an ambulance and within thirty minutes he had arrived at the hospital. A ruptured, or rupturing, aortic aneurysm, had been diagnosed and after cross-matching a bucket load of blood, he was anaesthetised and surgery began.

The operation had only one aim. To stop the bleeding and then replace the damaged aorta with a graft. But clamping the aorta and arresting the blood supply to the lower part of the body puts huge strain on the heart. Any unrecognised cardiac problem might lead to a heart attack or catastrophic cardiac rhythm change. Even though a smoker for fifty years, the patient was fairly fit. It was considered that he would get through the procedure. Anyway, there was no alternative.

When the surgeon opened the peritoneum, he recognised the aneurysm immediately. The large tense pulsating mass at the back of the abdomen. It was now beginning to leak into the wider abdominal cavity, filling the peritoneum with blood.

Within fifteen minutes of starting the operation, the aorta was clamped just below the renal arteries and at the lower end across both common iliac vessels. Through a vertical incision in the wall of the aorta, an enormous quantity of thrombus and atheroma (Greek athērē = porridge) was scooped out by the gloved hand of the surgeon. It had the consistency of thick porridge. Ali, the vascular surgeon, was a well-established consultant and knew exactly what he was doing. A substantial amount of blood was seen back-bleeding from the lumbar vessels that supplied the spine via the back of the aorta. These were quickly under-run with sutures.

Now the surgeon was ready to begin sewing in the aortic graft. Made of polyethylene terephthalate, a durable polyester, and marketed under the name of 'Dacron', Ali trimmed down the pre-packed sterile tube he had been given by his scrub nurse to about 12 centimetres in length. That would be enough to bridge the gap where the aorta had been leaking. Now all that was left of the aneurysm was a floppy sac and a big hole into which to place the graft. Ali knew that this inert material was durable and would never need replacing during his patient's lifetime.

With a diameter of only about three centimetres this Dacron cylindrical graft is made up of firm white material with the consistency of cloth. It is able to expand in length considerably as the corrugations built into it can be stretched under tension. Ali knew that he must sew in place just the right length of graft. Too long and it would kink upwards. Too short and it would put the sutures in the fragile remaining aorta under too much tension and they would give way.

He began the careful business of stitching in the graft using a moderately fine but strong nylon suture. First he sewed in the posterior aspect and then with a continuous suture technique all the way round the front as well. It was a procedure he had carried out a hundred times or more. When completed he let off the clamp and a jet of blood confirmed the upstream end was patent and the join was not bleeding very much. Ali then turned his attention to the lower end and began sewing that in.

It was at the moment he was completing that task that he realised that this operation was not going to be complication free.

'I am losing pressure Ali. Is anything bleeding?' shouted the anaesthetist.

'Bit of oozing from the upstream end only, John. Can I take off the iliac clamps and perfuse his legs now?'

'Wait until I get this unit of blood into him, please! I think he may have a pump problem. He has gone into fast AF!'

'OK! I will wait,' said Ali calmly. 'Sister, could your runner send out a message to the coffee room for Catherine to come into theatre, please.'

Catherine was the senior vascular surgeon in the unit. As she hurried to Theatre 9, she was thinking how vascular surgery had changed over the years. Open surgery using big incisions was not as common as it once was. This was due to the arrival of stenting and the EVAR technique, endovascular repair. This minimally invasive method inserts an internal support to bolster the aorta's crumbling architecture. The stent, in collapsed form, is passed in a catheter from one of the femoral arteries in the groin. This avoids much of the trauma of the open surgery that needs a large abdominal incision. It is then expanded in place by releasing it from the catheter. It cannot solve every problem and comes with problems of its own. It cannot always be applied to the emergency cases but it has a growing part to play in the treatment of these aneurysms both in the aorta and in other parts of the vascular tree.

***

Ali and Catherine had been asked to operate together for the open cases as they were now becoming considerably rarer. They had both had a run of poor outcomes in the last few months which is not unusual, as was illustrated at the beginning of this chapter. In consequence the medical director had asked them to carry out their cases together.

Ali had interpreted this advice as making sure he was in the hospital when Catherine was operating and vice versa. Being on hand in the coffee room seemed close enough and Catherine had interpreted this new rule from the medical director similarly.

'Hi Catherine! Thanks for popping into theatre. Seems that on releasing the proximal clamp this patient has had some kind of cardiac event. Not sure there was anything I could have done differently. Both anastomoses [the joins between the graft and the native vessel] are not bleeding much at all.'

At that moment John the anaesthetist called 'CARDIAC ARREST' and all hell broke loose.

It was not going to be a good day for anyone.

***

Every unexpected death, or death during or soon after an operation, is reported to the coroner. The death of Ali's patient followed this routine. The coroner advised the clinicians who had looked after him that a coroner's post-mortem would be arranged. In consequence they were unable to write a death certificate.

The government's own Guide to Coroner's Services for Bereaved People defines a coroner as:

'a special judge who investigates unnatural or violent deaths, where the cause of death is unknown, or because the death took place in prison, police custody or another type of state detention, such as a mental health hospital. It adds that the investigation may include an inquest hearing and that the coroner's role is to find out who died and how, when, and where they died.'

Most importantly as we will see to the contrary in Chapter 19:

'the coroner cannot make a finding that someone is guilty of something or to blame for something.'

A week later the whole process had been completed and a death certificate had been issued following the coroner's instructions:

Cause of Death: Ruptured Aortic Aneurysm
Contributing Factors: Ischaemic Heart Disease

A two weeks later the patient was cremated in a nearby crematorium.

***

On the same day the patient was cremated, both Ali and his senior colleague Catherine were summoned to the office of the new medical director of Northwick Park Hospital. This was an unusual step and both surgeons were nervous as they climbed the short flight of steps to Dr. David Woburn's office where he was slumped in a chair fiddling with his laptop. He was an ugly, rather fat fellow with a displeasing manner. After cursory handshakes and introductions to his assistant, who was also present, Dr. Woburn got down to business straightaway.

'Mr. Ali, following the death of your patient, who was admitted with a ruptured aneurysm on the 24th of October and who died the same day on the operating table, I am suspending you from all duties with immediate effect.'

'With regard your senior colleague Catherine, I am demanding that she carries out no more open vascular cases until my investigations are complete.'

For a few moments no-one in the room said anything.

'I demand also that you suspend all your private operating as well from this moment.'

All the colour had drained from Ali's face and Catherine was staring at the floor.

Finally Ali spoke.

'But I carried out the operation in a judicious manner without surgical complication. The fellow's heart just could not take the trauma of a rupture and then a repair with the concomitant clamping and re-perfusion injury that occurs when the clamps are released.'

'That may be the case but I specifically wrote to you both two months ago that these cases must be handled together.'

'But Catherine was in the operating theatre suite and as soon as it looked like there was going to be a problem I called her straight in to help.'

'But that is not what I demanded from you. In addition, for some time there have been rumours from some of your outpatient staff that you are late for clinics and early to leave the clinic in the sole charge of your registrars.'

Ali was stumped for words as the sharpness of these statements echoed round the medical director's large office.

'I believe that occasionally when you are due to work in the private sector you have been known to leave early. What do you say to that?'

'I do not think that has happened on more than a couple of occasions, Dr. Woburn, and for that I am sorry. But to suspend me from all duties over a case I handled perfectly correctly is a bit of an overkill, if you pardon the pun?'

Before Dr. Woburn could reply, Catherine spoke up firmly.

'I agree with Ali, Dr. Woburn. This suspension seems an unusually severe way to approach the inherent difficulties of vascular surgery.'

'Enough! I do not wish to hear any more about it. My decision stands and I am appointing an external surgeon to look at both your conducts. Now if both of you do not mind I have an important meeting with the chief executive starting in two minutes.'

Ali and Catherine walked slowly up the main corridor of the hospital mulling over what they had just heard. Ali began a stream of near-hysterical sentences.

'If I am suspended from Northwick Park can I carry on with any of my other practice? If I lose my private practice income I will not be able to pay the mortgage on my North London house. My wife has just had her second baby and her mother is ill back in India. What am I to say to her?'

Catherine kept her counsel. There were plenty of unhappy thoughts going round her head at the same time.

In fact, in the next three weeks Ali did not say much to his wife at all. He was too ashamed to admit to her that he had been suspended from the hospital so he just packed his golf clubs in the back of his car and spent all day on the fairways. Although it was not what he had planned, after a few days his handicap was improving significantly. This may have given him some satisfaction but it was no compensation from the shock he had received at the hands of Dr. Woburn.

When he enquired later for further clarification on paper as to why he had been suspended, he was told by the medical director's office that reasons could not be specified as it was all sub-judice and that he had not actually been 'suspended' just 'excluded' from the hospital. He was also informed that he should not continue working privately at this time. After two more attempts at contacting the medical director he was not much wiser.

'There had been a few complaints… about time-keeping… and clinical effectiveness…' was the only feedback he had received.

After a couple of weeks of this Ali telephoned me.

'Peter, you are the senior surgeon on the unit and I know you have an interest helping colleagues who get into difficulties. Can you help me?'

Ali told me the problem and the harsh way he had been treated by Dr. Woburn.

'Why did he need to be so sharp and unpleasant to a colleague?' Ali continued.

I detected he was nearly on the point of sobbing down the phone. Certainly he was not the normal bright, outgoing surgeon I knew. He had been with me on several hard four-day walks I had organised in the mountains of Scotland. I knew him to be a man of much energy and enthusiasm. He seemed now to be a shadow of the walker, squash player and surgeon that I knew he was.

I tried to console him.

'I do not know why these medical directors need to be as they are. They may get their enhanced pay and pension but they lose all our respect,'

I continued, thinking I had probably said too much.

'What do we know about Dr. Woburn, Peter? Where did he come from?' asked Ali.

'I have been doing some research on him since I got your call and spoke to one of his old bosses, an old chum of mine from medical school who is the senior physician at the hospital where he worked. He said that Dr. Woburn, who was his registrar ten years ago, was the laziest and rudest registrar he had ever had. He would never take responsibility for his own mistakes but would readily try and place the blame on others. My friend could not wait for him to rotate out of his service.'

'And now he's our medical director and torturing us.'

'Yes, but we have to learn to live with it. These people are very powerful,' I warned.

'Let's see how the independent enquiry goes.' I continued.

'Try and keep up your morale in the short-term. By the way, I am sure you are not obliged to give up your private work. Just tell the chief executives in those hospitals what is happening and they will almost certainly allow you to carry on.'

Ali did just that and was supported by the executive officers at the private sites where he worked. He kept his private practice going, at least in part. It meant he did not have to default on his mortgage and, finally a further week later, plucked up enough courage to tell his wife what had happened. She was as mystified as he was by the sudden turn of events. But she was relieved too as his odd behaviour had made her suspect that he might be having an affair with a woman, and not just a medical director.

The week before the independent enquiry was due to submit its report Ali suffered severe chest pain on the tenth green at his golf club. He was raced to Northwick Park Hospital where a heart attack, a myocardial infarct, was diagnosed. The angiogram showed a constricting lesion of one of his cardiac arteries and a cardiac stent was inserted across it.

After two nights in hospital he got back home to convalesce. Four days later he heard the news that the independent enquiry could see no wrongdoing in the actions of either Ali or Catherine. His suspension had been lifted and that he would be soon returning to work. The news of his reinstatement came through his secretary who had received a direct communication from Dr. Woburn's office by email only.

No conciliatory note.

No apology.

Nothing to suggest anyone other than a robot was ever involved.

His cardiologist too was delighted but would not hear of his patient resuming the stressful work of a vascular surgeon immediately.

'Not for at least six weeks, Ali. After what you have been through you are not to work until I tell you and that is all there is to be said about it,' he stated emphatically.

When Ali returned to work we convened a meeting of the Medical Staff Committee of which I had once been chairman. I decided to ask Dr. Woburn to attend as I wanted to emphasise to him how poorly I thought the consultant staff were being treated.

In times past the discipline of a hospital was enforced by a panel system of senior consultants who would look at a problem when it arose and discuss it with the doctor in question. This semi-formal arrangement was called The Three Wise Men committee. Today it would have to be The Three Wise Doctors, I suppose. These committees had been abolished thirty years ago. Politicians and managers had not liked the idea that senior experts were policing other experts.

I presented a paper to the fifty consultants who were attending the meeting. I titled my talk A Lament for the Three Wise Men (or Women). It detailed the manner of any investigation that follows an adverse clinical incident. I expressed how harshly nowadays these enquiries were being conducted.

'There is no need to always look for blame and bad motive when something goes wrong,' I argued.

'To suspend a perfectly able doctor for several weeks as if they were on remand for a serious crime is inappropriate. Especially as they are so often fully exonerated a couple of months later. It all causes such stress. In the end the doctor's morale is broken. I surmise that after such misery the doctor may want to find another organisation to work for. Even worse they may yearn for an early retirement or even leave the service immediately to go farming in Devon,' I continued.

'Why cannot we be disciplined by benign headmasters? Firm but kind. That should be the motto. Not vindictive inquisitors as it seemed in the case of Ali,' I concluded.

Dr. Woburn had been sitting awkwardly at the front of the room shifting the weight of his body from side to side and referring to his laptop. At this point he stood up and faced the audience.

'You do not seem to realise that I have to follow the guidance laid down in the Department of Health's Maintaining High Professional Standards. My duty is to the patients and their safety. I am not interested in the individual doctor and his or her morale. I have a duty of safeguarding and that is what I will do. In the case of Ali I would do the same again every time.'

There was general disquiet in the room, as it was quite clear that not one of the doctors present agreed with the medical director's philosophy. I kept up the fight by reminding Dr. Woburn that at Section 9.9 of the document that he was quoting to us it stated: 'Remedial action rather than solely disciplinary action must be considered...'

Dr. Woburn just reiterated his former stance and sat down gruffly.

Some started to leave the hall. Others pressed hard with some pertinent questions. After a few more unhelpful statements from Dr. Woburn we called the meeting to close.

***

After a decade at Northwick Park Hospital, I became a clinical director, responsible for the administration of the surgical services. It was well remunerated and I had a general feeling that it was a good thing to do to support the hospital in that way. It might also help me receive Merit points. And points mean prizes! Now called ACCEA points, these extra payments are valuable. Consultants can even double their salary and their pension if they are outstanding. These rare individuals may receive a Platinum Award. They would normally have to be internationally or nationally recognised to reach this level. Most of us aspire to somewhere well below that lofty label.

These awards were developed deliberately to encourage salaried consultants to do additional work in research, teaching, national administration or local management. With this aim they have largely achieved their goals. Climbing up the ladder of these award points is a slow business but one of the quickest ways is to go into medical management and become a medical director or an assistant director. It may be a lot easier than having to develop a clinical or scientific research team, pioneer new treatments or run a national medical organisation. In consequence it does not necessarily attract the most brilliant.

Of course, running any organisation takes skill and time. It requires much patience and persistence. When I ran the Department of Surgery, it was a difficult task trying to balance budgets, appoint staff, motivate those already in place, and innovate. Change was always very slow. I felt often it was like swimming in treacle. It was difficult to get much done. I would attend hospital board meetings and go to management seminars where platitudes and long lists of good intentions were repeated like mantras. These meetings had their own management-speak language often used to deliberately obscure the common sense needed to be applied to a problem. When there was an elephant in the room this was never acknowledged.

In the NHS today no member of staff can escape management's bureaucratic tentacles. New directives from on high make everyone compulsorily attend courses, often on the latest politically sensitive topic. It is almost like following fashion trends. Training is now needed in disability, racism, safeguarding, consent, mental capacity, breaking bad news, terrorism prevention, patient lifting, infection control, fire prevention, and much more besides.

At one point I was obliged to attend an afternoon course on 'Conducting a Medical Consultation'.

Along with ten other surgeons, I was lectured to by a young man just out from university with a second-class psychology degree. As I looked around the room at my colleagues' incredulous faces, I was struck by the stupidity of this exercise. I calculated that these men and women had conducted more than one and a half million patient consultations between them. Many encounters would have been simple but some were very complex involving the passing of very bad news. Here we were all listening to a well-meaning twenty-three year old who had never performed such a task but had read the theory in a psychology textbook.

The modern world of management we have created is often bizarre and illogical. I think the rot started in earnest in the US in the late 1970s in some business school. It seems it has since spread across the globe inexorably. I often think of it as an unstoppable management virus for which there is no known cure.

After five years in the post of clinical director my appetite to progress higher up the management ladder in the NHS was exhausted. I stepped aside and passed the post on to a younger and more eager colleague. But again and again over the years I have been struck how these positions of authority are misused. Having been part of the system for a short while, I am the first to acknowledge that running anything, a hospital, a company, a government, is not an easy thing to do. But the way organisations now approach it is all wrong.

I keep coming back to the concept of the good headmaster.

When I was seven years old I went to a school where the headmaster was amusing, liberal-minded and wanted us to thrive by both working and playing hard. He made sure we all had a lot of fun. In consequence, he was much loved and the pupils would do anything for him. And they did. They strived for excellence and the results reflected this. But at the same time as fostering this liberal, fair-minded approach that same headmaster was firm. When discipline was needed he applied it resolutely but never in the churlish, resentful, holier-than-thou, angry, unfair way that seems to be the norm today.

Too often I have seen the vision of self-importance on the faces of these medical managers. Like a pompous examiner torturing a student in an examination, they flaunt their positions from a position of strength. One of my long-time surgical colleagues at the hospital became the medical director in his final three years before retiring. From being a sharp, rather joyless but very effective and respected clinician, he became a pious bully who was much feared, even loathed.

By the time he retired he had lost most of his friends.

**

Ali is now back at work at Northwick Park Hospital. He has had not had a recurrence of his heart problem and is playing golf with a better handicap score and hitting a squash ball as vigorously as his fifty-something years will allow. But he has decided to avoid, as far as possible, the high risk surgery that led him to be so criticised that day. Now he is meticulous with his time-keeping and will often ask a colleague advice with a difficult case.

This may be good for his mental health but by the same measure a lot of the joy in his work seems to have left him. He plods on month by month avoiding the managers as far as he can while secretly planning his retirement. He even applied for a job elsewhere but was not successful.

If he does retire early and before his time, I will remind him to turn the lights off at Northwick Park Hospital because, if the Soviet-style management system continues to terrorise consultants, as it does in many hospitals up and down our land, all his colleagues will have already retired before him.

An empty shell of a hospital needs no lights burning.

But it is time to think happier thoughts with the help of those wonderful souls I have had the privilege to treat all of my working life – children.

Chapter 17:
Little People And Small Incisions

❖

There is a famous painting by Edvard Munch, the Norwegian painter, with the title The Sick Child. It is the image of his fifteen-year-old older sister dying of tuberculosis in 1877. Only the most hardened heart could not be moved by this depiction of the unfairness of being selected to die so young.

When I was a very young doctor I toyed with entering into many specialties other than surgery but they all had their drawbacks. A physician treats only adults, a psychiatrist could be frustrated by his patients' lack of progress, a tropical medicine consultant may be obliged to travel continuously and might catch a whole raft of diseases himself, while an obstetrician and gynaecologist is obliged to treat only women. At least as a general surgeon I would be entitled to treat men, women and children. That for me was one of surgery's attractions.

Although I have treated children as a general surgeon all my working life, I have been mostly spared the anguish and pain that Munch's painting conjures up. Most of the children I treat are fit and happy with solvable problems. If I had become a paediatric oncologist, as one of my musician friends became, treating children with cancer and blood disorders, I am sure the painting of The Sick Child would be in my mind often as I watched some of my patients die. Of course, there would be moments of happiness to compensate for the distress of observing such misery. Many children would be cured of their terrible tumours but it would still be very hard at times.

My line of work as a part-time paediatric general surgeon operating on children has almost always been easy and is carried out in children with a normal life expectancy. I can make most a bit better. I was lucky enough in 1983 as a young surgeon to do a year as a registrar in the Children's Hospital in Southampton. A well-recognised paediatric unit, it was well run and had high standards. It was managed, as most paediatric units are, by people with a calling to be kind, cheerful and nice. Indeed these doctors, paediatric physicians, psychiatrists and surgeons, often possess a self-conviction which amounts almost to religious faith. I understand this. After all, what could be more important in the world than treating little people with their trusting eyes, their exquisite vulnerability, their extraordinary sense of humour and their long lives ahead of them.

Almost as important is the fact that treating kids is fun. With few exceptions they are so happy and so easily cheered. Like puppies they laugh and play a lot. They are always inquisitive and their language is hysterically funny. You can almost see them changing their perception of the world by the hour. Their bodies mostly do not bear the scars of time and only a small proportion are grossly overweight. This last fact for a surgeon who operates often on obese adults is a rare treat.

But when I was working in Southampton I noticed something odd about children. We adults had our own language laid out in dictionaries while the children had their own vocabulary, which was not. It was like talking Spanish to a Frenchman. It did not always work. When I wanted to know if they had vomited or had their bowels open I could not quite find the right words. I would have to experiment quite a lot to get the little person to understand. Naturally, I could ask the parents to help but that immediately compounded the problem by talking through a third party.

Like trying to communicate with an adult who cannot understand you, an interpreter can aid the exchange but there is always a barrier to comprehension. In addition this secret language that I had discovered was very different in the youngest children compared with the adolescents. The words that a three-year old might use would be entirely distinct from that used by a fourteen-year old. So much so that I was always trying to find the right words to use for the right child.

It was exhausting.

I had the idea that I might be able to unlock these language codes so devised a study which might help me do just that. I surveyed a hundred children with their parents asking them to tell me what common words they used for some of the bodily functions of interest to me as a general surgeon. Naturally, when you treat the guts, the groins, the bottom, and the genitalia the language becomes quite agricultural so I had to warn the parents of my frankness. In the process there were quite a lot of laughs on the way. One hundred children from two to fifteen years of age took part in the study.

I took eight words. I wanted to know the commonest used words to express some delicate anatomical parts such as penis, vagina, anus and testicles and physiological functions such as defaecation, anal flatulence, micturition (passing urine) and vomiting. Such is the language of a surgeon who fixes groin problems and the guts.

The results were both enlightening and amusing. For penis (14) willy (36), winkle (4), widgie (4) and dinkle (3) were common while for vagina (6) fanny (14), pinkie (1), tweet (1), fluffy bit (1), front bottom (1), tuppenny (1) and ninny (1) were used. Anus was called bum (46) by nearly half of the group with bottom (29), arse (3) and backside (1) featuring, while testicles (10) was not commonly understood – with seventy-six children answering 'don't know' - but balls (10), stones (1), goalies (1), privates (1), nuts (1) and rugby balls (1) were occasionally used.

Defaecation was pooh (48) in nearly half with loo (8), plops (3) and number two (2) being used less often while anal flatulence was fart (29), a pardon (10), wind (6), blow off (6), fluffed (5), permped (4) or bum burp (3). Micturition or urination was easy with wee wee (61), toilet (21) and loo (7), and vomiting was sick (67) with only puke (4) and throw up (2) being used by the adolescents.

There were a lot of idiosyncratic words developed by families which made the findings particularly interesting. Some were too rude to be repeated. Others were just plain silly.

Armed with these results I wrote a paper entitled Favourite Words and sent it to the most prestigious paediatric journal in the land, The Archives of Diseases of Childhood. Much to the envy of my full-time paediatric medical colleagues it was published to some acclaim.

Although it was a bit of fun there was a serious intention to it. I hoped it would help paediatricians and surgeons communicate better with their little patients.

**

In my early years at Northwick Park we performed emergency surgery even on babies. I had written a paper from Basingstoke District Hospital ten years before on the subject of congenital hypertrophic pyloric stenosis, affectionately known as 'pi'. I had demonstrated that treating these babies in a district hospital was just as safe as sending them to a specialist paediatric surgical unit. This curious condition of pi is quite common and oddly affects male to female babies by four to one. It is also more common in first born infants.

Excessive vomiting of milk feeds begins about four to six weeks after birth in an otherwise healthy baby. The vomiting is fierce and is described as projectile. I remember examining one such baby when he vomited. Unlike my experience in Accident & Emergency described in Chapter 5, on this occasion I was quick enough to duck my head as the vomited feed hit the nurse standing behind me.

This vomiting is due to the fact that the pylorus, or outflow channel from the stomach to the duodenum, has become thickened and milk cannot pass easily. No-one knows why. Could it be a virus, a constituent of milk or a hereditary defect as you are more likely to be afflicted if your twin has it? Luckily for me as an identical twin my brother did not develop it though I do monitor him carefully for other diseases even today.

It took until the first part of the twentieth century for an operation to be developed that would safely cure this condition. Before that time many babies died of dehydration without surgery and many others following the major surgical procedures advised at the time. A German surgeon named Wilhelm Ramstedt from Münster in 1911 decided simply to fillet the thickened muscle of the pylorus longitudinally to release the pressure.

Miraculously not only is the obstruction immediately relieved but the condition almost never recurs and there are no long term side effects. Once Ramstedt had shown his little operation's safety and efficacy, it became the standard. Mostly performed through a three centimetre incision above the tummy button it can now be carried out with tiny incisions and mini-laparoscopic instruments.

When I first arrived at Northwick Park Hospital, I was referred these babies often as I was known to have an interest. Despite this there were not that many cases to see. I operated maybe on four or five a year. It has been said that surgical patients, like buses, sometimes come in threes. I recall a Friday night in 1992 when I diagnosed one baby with this condition at lunchtime, another by teatime and yet another just before I had supper. That night I had a confident children's anaesthetist with me and our emergency list became a production line. Three in one long evening. A record.

I am glad to say that all the babies did well.

We also used to do operations on children who presented with the second most difficult word in medicine to spell, 'intussusception'. Actually, the most difficult word to spell is the almost unmentionable 'epididymis', which lies behind the testis. Intussusception (Latin - *intus* within and *suscipere* to receive) is when the intestine pushes into the part below, appearing to be trying to expel itself. The bowel wall swells and the result is obstruction. This phenomenon is seen very occasionally in an adult when a tumour or a polyp is mistaken for a bolus of stool and peristalsis tries unsuccessfully to push it through. But in infants between three and nine months it is much more common even in what appears to be normal intestine. It is not really known why this should happen but the babies arrive with colicky pain, redcurrant jelly stools, a sausage-shaped lump and finally obstruction and rarely perforation.

Someone had the bright idea that blowing saline or air up the bottom of these mites under the right pressure might reduce the intussusception. Miraculously it worked in over half the cases and it does not recur often. Those that do not benefit from this insufflation method need an operation to remove the segment and I did quite a few in those early years.

Operating on children is a pleasure. It seems perverse to state that fact but the tissues are small and perfect. It is intricate work but as children heal so quickly the complications commonly seen in adults with their poorer arterial blood supply are very rare in children.

Nowadays these abdominal operations in the UK have largely been centralised as paediatric surgery has developed. General surgeons like me, who were trained adequately in basic paediatric surgery, are rare now in the modern health service. Also anaesthetists outside the paediatric hospitals are less confident performing anaesthetics on babies than they use to be.

I suppose that means I am now irreplaceable. That feels nice but before I get carried away and my head swells, I must always remind myself of that poem that begins:

One day when you're feeling important
One day when your ego's in bloom
One day when you think you are
The most important man in the room…

And ends after five verses:

The moral of this is quite simple
Be true to yourself and just do the best that you can
But always remember
There's no irreplaceable man!

***

I hinted that an operation as simple as Ramstedt's procedure for the thickened outflow to the stomach in babies is now also being carried out by the keyhole method using tiny instruments. Probably there is not much benefit over the open method except that the scars, usually three five-millimetre scars, are tiny. Although the scar with the open method is not much bigger than the end of a lumberjack's thumb when the operation is completed, unfortunately scars in children grow as a child grows. They become quite disfiguring sometimes. So maybe there is a clear cosmetic advantage if the holes are smaller.

Laparoscopic surgery as I touched upon in Chapter 9 was pioneered by gynaecologists to inspect tubes and ovaries. However, by the early 1990s general surgeons had adapted it to remove appendixes, gall-bladders, colons and even fix hernias. There was an explosion in new equipment. Computer chip TV cameras and video imaging facilitated the images and the ability both to teach and to share the images. Recordings could be made and the image sent down a phone line to a distant place.

This was not the end of it. So-called robots were brought into the equation, allowing the surgeon to control the long key-hole instruments away from the operating table while sitting at a comfortable console. Awkward movements of hands could be ironed out as the machines allow for extra degrees of movement while the monitors offer improved images.

The console for the robots is usually in the same operating theatre as the patient but they do not have to be. It is now possible for a surgeon in New York to perform an operation in Paris. This was done to great applause some years ago, though it took France Telecom three months' work to set up the electronics to do it. Today I think it might take thirty minutes and a good computer expert to arrange.

We now have highly trained surgeons using robots to remove rectums, prostate glands and much else besides. It all takes a bit more time but a lot more money. The machines alone cost £1 million and the disposables used for each patient many thousands of pounds. But the patients seem to benefit from the high precision these operations afford.

Needless to say, it was the younger surgeons who could see these advantages as they were introduced and whose more supple minds could learn the techniques easily. Although I had long since learnt to take gall bladders out successfully with the laparoscope, I only dabbled in the more advanced techniques required for removing large organs like the colon. I judged it was time to pass on the baton to the young.

Only fools do not know that they will one day be surpassed by those coming after them. Us late-adopters, as we are called now, are never really irreplaceable as in the poem. I could see that quite clearly but others that do not see this sometimes made big mistakes in pursuing new techniques they could not master.

It is a sign of maturity to recognise that the student will often overtake the teacher. So after twenty-three years at Northwick and St. Mark's Hospital, I opted to pass my colorectal cancer patients to these young thrusters and take a back seat doing the simpler, less glamorous procedures. In any discipline there is plenty of routine work to be done, which is usually less attractive to the young who want to be at the coalface where the cut and thrust of surgery is taking place.

I look now with pride at some of those that I have trained who now are pioneering these new operations. I look back and see myself thirty years ago where they are now. At the forefront. Some of these surgeons are so gifted that I am perpetually astonished. At first, it is hard to let others take over but it is the right thing to do as both the boldness and energy that we have when we are young, wears thin as time passes.

Someone asked me recently whether I had lost manual dexterity as I have aged. I answered that I had not lost dexterity but that I had lost my audacity. I envy those who buck this trend but they are few and far between.

***

Let me illustrate this new surgical world by comparing these new Titans of robotic surgery with the first known resection of a cancer of the rectum by the Parisian surgeon Jacques Lisfranc in 1826. Less than two centuries have passed between his time and ours.

Lisfranc's patient was operated on from below with an incision around the anus and by blunt dissection to mobilise the rectum. Then the surgeon amputated it high up inside the pelvis. Lisfranc then crudely sewed up the upper rectum and formed a colostomy in the abdominal wall on the lower left side.

Opium, in the form of laudanum, would have been administered as an oral elixir before the operation. Lisfranc could have obtained some nitrous oxide from England to put the patient to sleep for it had been described previously in 1800 by Humphrey Davy. But I doubt he did that as it was overlooked as an anaesthetic agent until the end of the nineteenth century. Ether and chloroform were not discovered until a little later so the poor patient only had a bit of Cognac to add to the opium.

What is clear is that the patient would have suffered agonies during Lisfranc's smash and grab to remove the rectum. He would have been held down by four strong orderlies and strapped firmly to the operating table. A large crowd of interested observers would be present. Just like Lisfranc they would be wearing their usual frock coats stained with blood from previous operations.

Lisfranc's initial incision would have created a very small, dark space high in the pelvis with blood pouring out of it. Using fairly basic instruments and with silk or catgut sutures Lisfranc might have attempted to secure bleeding vessels if he could actually see them. When that attempt failed the cavity would have been packed vigorously with thick gauze to stop the haemorrhage. Sometimes it worked but often it would not stop and the patient would bleed to death. Taking the gauze out of the cavity five days later would have been another agony. Post-operatively the colostomy would be a nightmare for the patient. No bags. Just control the effluent with rags.

Lisfranc proudly reported his first nine cases. Three died. All had permanent colostomies as no surgeon dared to rejoin the bowel at that time. Nothing is known of the long-term outcome of his patients but within a year most of the patients' tumours would have recurred after which they would have died unpleasantly in great pain.

***

Now let us compare that with the ritual of a robotic-assisted resection of the rectum carried out in the year 2021.

Pre-operatively the patient is briefed fully and consented. Blood is taken to prepare for transfusion on the rare chance it is needed. Bowels are prepared with purgatives to allow a cleaner field and reduce post-operative sepsis. The patient is anaesthetised via a tiny canula in his arm and then knows nothing of the rest of the procedure. He is given a large dose of morphine (from opium) intravenously, nitrous oxide and oxygen to inhale and a full muscle relaxant to aid the surgery. He is usually given other inhalation anaesthetic agents to aid anaesthesia. Antibiotics are administered to reduce post-operative infection.

The patient already has an epidural catheter in place dripping some bupivacaine, a local anaesthetic, into that space near the spinal cord resulting in almost complete lack of sensation and allowing the intravenous analgesics to be reduced to safer levels. A small dose of heparin has been given to reduce post-operative venous thrombosis and the patients legs are wrapped and intermittently compressed by pumps to keep the circulation going.

The abdomen is prepped and toweled up by the surgeon and the tiny incisions for the laparoscopic instruments made. The instruments are inserted carefully under direct vision guided by images on the high definition TV screens. All of the individuals close to the patient are gowned, masked and gloved and all is done under the strictest sterile conditions. The air in the operating theatre is fully recirculated ten times an hour to reduce the chance of airborne infection. The laparoscopic instruments are 'docked' into the control arm of the robot. There are dissecting instruments, energy sources such as ultrasonic or diathermy dissectors and the operation commences.

The surgeon sits at the console and may even take a coffee while he operates. He or she calls for the patient to be tilted on the table, left, right, feet up, head down to allow the small intestine to fall out of the pelvis and give him a good view of the rectum. The tumour is large and visible on the front of the rectum and the dissection begins. Meticulously the surgeon develops the plane behind the rectum and includes all the nodes and blood vessels in the mesentery as they may carry tumour.

There is no bleeding at all as any vessel that even threatens to bleed is quickly closed by using one of his heat source instruments or occasionally a clip. It takes a while but the surgeon makes certain that the tumour is resected with a good margin of normal tissue around it to make local tumour recurrence less likely. The position of the table is changed with the patient, who is securely held in position, placed at a twenty-degree tilt to the right while the left colon is mobilised. This allows the colon to reach the lower rectum for later join-up. The assistant surgeon who is standing at the operating theatre with the scrub nurse assists in the next few moves.

A 60 millimetre laparoscopic stapling device with two lines of staples and a knife is fired mechanically below the tumour closing off the rectum and sealing the upper end so that no contents can escape. The tumour and rectum are extracted from a small incision through a plastic sleeve or 'wound excluder' to avoid contamination of the wound with live cancer cells or bacteria. A linear cutter is passed across the colon above the rectum and the specimen removed through a small incision and sent for analysis by an expert pathologist. The end of the colon is passed back into the pelvis after the head of a circular stapling device, the 'gun', has been sewn into it. The CO_2 gas, which has provided the distention during the operation, is pumped in once more. The 'gun' is passed up the anus and joins up with the head and then fired.

The colon has been perfectly joined to the lower rectum.

No tension.

Good blood supply.

No mess.

The whole surgical field is checked for bleeding. There have only been 20 millilitres of blood spilled during the whole three-hour procedure. Miraculous. The chances of post-operative complications are low.

The robotic arm is undocked and the laparoscopic instruments removed. The wounds are carefully sutured. Local anaesthetic, which was not introduced to surgery until 1884, is injected liberally into the wounds to reduce post-operative discomfort. The patient is allowed to wake up. There is some abdominal and shoulder discomfort but a further shot of morphine blunts this quite quickly.

'Have I had the operation?' The patient asks in the recovery suite.

'Yes, you have Mr. Smith. Do you feel any pain?'

'I feel nauseous and bit bloated but not much real pain.'

'On a scale of ten what is your pain?'

'About a three at the moment, I would say.'

'In your right hand is a button. When you need it just press it and you will get a little top up for the pain.'

'Can I phone my wife?'

'Yes, of course. And by the way the cancer has been fully removed and the surgeon says he is very pleased with how the operation has gone. It took a time to do well but that damned tumour is well and truly history.'

'What a relief! Thank you, nurse.'

The patient goes back to the ward and is given a cup of tea four hours later. Food is given the next day as well as high calorie and protein drinks. The patient mobilises early and is discharged seventy-two hours later to recover at home.

**

How different the experience is today compared with that of Lisfranc's patients. Although we cannot ask any of that great French surgeon's patients to appear as witness to the agonies they suffered, we do have a first-hand account from novelist Charles Dickens when he had his fistula-in-ano operated upon at St. Mark's. Dickens was known to have a jaundiced attitude towards the medical profession and their institutions but there is no reason for us to question the veracity of his statements made after his operation had been completed:

'last Friday morning I was obliged to submit to a cruel operation, and the cutting out root and branch of a disease caused by working over much which has been gathering it seems for years…

I suffered agonies, as they related all to me, and did violence to myself in keeping to my seat. I could scarcely bear it...

All manner of queer pains were floating about my illustrious person...'

And this was the great novelist's reaction to a minor peri-anal operation.

We can only imagine what he might have written if he had needed his rectum removed.

***

I began this chapter by relating how paediatric surgery has been a small but significant part of my surgical experience and finished it relating the modern method of performing a major resection of the rectum through tiny incisions.

In just two hundred years surgery has moved from darkness to light.

From inflicting agony to curing dangerous diseases in a civilised, almost pain-free manner.

None of this would have been possible without our anaesthetic colleagues.

This chapter should, by rights, be dedicated to them.

I have worked with many fine ones.

I will always be grateful for the skill with which they administer their mysterious medicines that allow surgeons like me to work at our ease while our patients sleep.

***

All the advances illustrated in this chapter came about from decade upon decade of medical research by young men and women in dozens of countries. My own efforts in this field have been very modest. But forty-five years ago I now recall I contributed a little.

Chapter 18:
A Journey To The USA

❖

It was the summer of 1985. I was standing in a beach bar on the island of Rhodes in the Eastern Aegean. The late afternoon Greek sun was still strong and the beer was cold and slightly sweet. That same morning I had given a paper at a surgical conference on the subject of sepsis in surgery. Having just completed a couple of years full-time research on the subject, I was somewhat of an authority on the topic at that moment in time.

The paper had been well received and I was feeling pleased with myself. I was ready for a bit of downtime, as the Americans say. As I stood gazing out to sea I noticed a famous English surgeon walking along the beach towards me. He had abandoned the UK for the USA many years before and had achieved fame and a bit of fortune on the other side of the pond.

The idea of working in America had been growing in my mind for a year or two and here was a chance to make it happen.

'Hello, Dr. Jagelman' I shouted. 'Fancy a beer?'

He obviously recognised me for he smiled and ambled to the bar.

'Sure, thanks. But I'm buying, OK?'

'If you insist,' I replied.

'It's Peter isn't it? I enjoyed your paper hugely. You were right to emphasise the misuse of antibiotics in surgery. They have a place but should not be overdone or we will see bacterial resistance growing even faster than it is already.'

'Thank you for your appreciation,' I replied.

There was an awkward pause as the beers arrived and Dr. Jagelman paid. I plucked up enough courage to ask the great man a favour.

'I was hoping to spend some time in the States and wondered if you might have any openings at the Cleveland Clinic?'

'Hmm! Why not? What would you want to research if you came over for a while?' he asked.

'Maybe some aspect of Crohn's disease if I could?'

He took a puff from his ever present cigarette. The bad habit that would kill him indirectly only a decade later.

'Well, we have so much inflammatory bowel disease at the clinic that you will find much to get your teeth into. Yeah! That would be fine. Although I am not much involved with Crohn's research these days I am certain Victor, the chief of colorectal surgery, would be happy to supervise you. I am sure you and he could write a few papers together.'

'Can I come over in August next year for six months, maybe?'

'No problem. Fix it with my secretary. We can pay you a modest stipend. It'll be nice having you over.'

Suddenly the beer tasted twice as good. As the sun began to sink in the west, I pressed my acquaintance for more information about the second largest hospital in the world.

***

So began my American adventure.

It would be something to look forward to. As soon as I returned home I began planning and less than a year later I found myself on a Northwest Orient jet bound for Cleveland, Ohio.

The immigration agent at the airport stopover in Boston looked at me and smiled sarcastically.

'Cleveland, Ohio, huh! You sure can't be going there for a vacation.'

It was a reaction that I heard again and again when people learnt of my destination in the States. Finally as the plane descended over Lake Erie I caught my first glance of the city. A clutch of skyscrapers, a thin film of sulphurous haze masquerading as a sunset, a messy network of freeways, a city divided by the Cuyahoga river, empty zones close to the downtown area where heavy industry had once brought great prosperity but were now no-go areas, and beyond all this mile upon mile of leafy suburbs.

I had arrived in the USA.

The land of extremes.

In the next few months I was to meet some of the kindest, rudest, ugliest, most beautiful, thinnest and fattest people I had ever seen in my life.

It was a warm evening as I walked out of the airport building. I suppose I was dressed like an Englishman because the chief of surgery's physician's assistant spotted me immediately.

'Is that Dr. Peter McDonald?'

The long American nasal drawl and the open vowels rang in my ears.

'Hi, I'm Beth! Lovely to meet you. Sorry! I cannot carry your bags as I have just had plastic surgery.'

Only in the USA would either statement, about my luggage or her recent surgery, be normal discourse.

Yes, I had arrived in the New World.

Beth was very cheerful and exceptionally friendly. She had kindly arranged for me to stay at her place for a day or two until I fixed up some permanent accommodation. We drove in her Ford Pinto towards the eastern suburbs of the city. She was indeed a hospitable hostess for within an hour of landing in Ohio I was sitting with Beth and a friend in her hot-tub under the stars drinking a California Merlot.

Living the American dream.

At 8am the next morning I checked into the Cleveland Clinic. It boasted that it was the second biggest hospital in the world with seven thousand five hundred employees. Half of the workers seemed to be involved in administration and its bureaucracy efficiently processed the newcomer on his first day. I was advised of my insurance, my health cover, given a badge and put on the payroll. My car park slot was pencilled electronically into my ID card. I was introduced to an accommodation agency and shown how to weigh my salad for payment at the staff canteen.

Surprisingly I was paid for the remainder of August on my fourth day and by the end of the week I had in my possession a mountain of glossy literature about the clinic. It stated boastfully that it was a national referral centre and an international health resource.

I got familiar with the clinic's four star hotel and met some of its own police force who ferried me between the buildings as the clinic was situated in a pretty dangerous part of the city. I shopped in its own huge supermarket and bought a few things from its very own massive drugstore. These retail outlets now are familiar to hospital visitors in the UK today, but they were unheard of in those days.

As I walked along the corridors outside the Department of Colorectal Surgery my feet tripped up on the thick Berber carpets lining the air conditioned skyways. I had to keep reminding myself that this was not a Hilton hotel or the VIP section of Riyadh International Airport but a so-called non-profit hospital in which I was to research the unpleasant, but slightly mysterious condition of Crohn's disease.

I was now a long way from that beach bar in Rhodes.

Far from home and the ancient, run-down NHS hospital in Southampton that I was accustomed to.

**

My life in Ohio quickly fell into a routine.

I found a bedroom in Shaker Heights just a twenty minute drive from the hospital. I lived in the attic room of a childless elderly African American couple. They were both retired and had plenty of time to tell me about the country from their point of view. Learning about the USA from a couple whose great grandparents had been slaves was enlightening. It was a good education.

One Sunday they took me to their Baptist Church where the hymns were sung loudly with many hallelujahs, much clapping and with the swaying of hips. I was the only white man there and many asked me if I was the driver of the coach that was waiting in the car park outside.

My work in the hospital was with a different tribe, many from overseas. The Chief of Colorectal Surgery, Victor Fazio, was a famous Australian surgeon. He was a workaholic. He would give a paper in Europe one day and fly back to the clinic during the night to spend fourteen hours operating, only to fly out again at midnight. Although he was a man running on tobacco and adrenaline, he was a kind fellow and set me off cutting up specimens of small intestine, which I collected from the operating theatre and took down to the professor of pathology for analysis.

It all worked out pretty well. By the end of my time in Cleveland I had written a few seminal articles, given some papers at a couple of American meetings in Los Angeles and New Orleans, and developed a theory about the pathology of the condition. Worthwhile from the point of view of my research but my main interest in being there was to observe the life and culture of the American health care system and to explore the country.

***

'I absolutely refuse to start my morning ward round before five o'clock in the morning,' said a fourth-year resident in general surgery to me one day.

An English listener unfamiliar with the USA would probably think he was raving mad. But he was deadly serious. Like most of the surgical residents or trainees he began every morning between 5am and 5.30am with an early ward round of his patients conducted without nurses. By 7am he had been round the patients under his care before meeting for the staff surgeon's round. After that was completed he went rushing to theatre or to the outpatient department. When his work there was finished he would see the new admissions and tidy up any loose ends before getting home any time between 8pm and 10pm.

A gruelling schedule indeed.

His job was looking after forty-five patients in the clinic. All were being fed intravenously as they had short gut syndrome and could not keep up their nutrition without help. Many of these were Crohn's sufferers in whom I had an interest.

Another evening I took a resident (registrar), Susan Galandiuk, a good talker and a very bright woman, into the bar in the clinic's hotel. She explained the system of training in the USA. It was different from the do-it-yourself training I had grown up with in the UK. The young American surgeons fight for the best training jobs and work flat out for five years, rotating every three months through all the specialties of surgery until they specialise with a year or two in a sub-specialty like colorectal surgery.

This had brought her to the Cleveland Clinic.

She would in the years to come go on to be a professor of surgery and a national figure in the subject.

In recent years we in the UK have begun to mirror the American system with its high university tuition fees and so-called run through training of the specialist. But when I looked at these surgical residents in Ohio they were exhausted and slightly cheerless. It is true that they were looking forward to earning good money after finishing their training in order to pay off the huge loans they had taken out to fund their studies and training. But the excessive workload came at quite a social cost to them.

While I was in Ohio, the only doctors I had a belly laugh with were ex-pats from Australia, New Zealand and the UK.

I got drunk with them too.

***

Although the Cleveland Clinic styled itself a not-for-profit organisation, this was a fib on a grand scale. It appeared to me that there was not a soul in America who did not think of money most of the time. It seemed to be in the air or maybe it was in the drinking water. Working at the second largest independent hospital in the world after the Mayo Clinic in Minnesota, money was very much part of the agenda. The patients were vetted for means of payment well before admission. Some were covered by Medicare and Medicaid, the old and the poor, while others were sponsored by work-related insurance, by voluntary schemes or simply paid in cash.

It was clear to me that the hospital did not want to see those that did not have the means to pay. I used to joke that the rather small Accident & Emergency Department of the Cleveland Clinic had the arrows pointing the wrong way. The clinic would much rather emergency patients went to Case Western in the centre of the city. The clinic would rather not be bothered with their urgent problems as they would interfere with the routines of the patients already scheduled and funded who came from all over the North American continent and beyond.

Hand-in-hand with checking that the patients had the means to pay comes the marketing of hospitals in the USA. Professional in the extreme it works at fever pitch. Competition is fierce and is tackled head on. At the Cleveland Clinic the Department of Public Affairs, as the marketing department is euphemistically called, had only four staff in 1980. By the time I arrived in1986 they employed one hundred and eight staff and its director was seen as very important for the clinic's survival.

How many would there be today in 2021?

There are advantages in this hard-nosed business approach. Innovation and research, which may bring kudos followed by patients into the hospital, is encouraged and is warmly rewarded. Good research brings fame and fame is its own generator of success. This is not the case in the NHS where innovations are difficult to introduce as they bring costs and stretch limited budgets.

The overcapacity of hospital facilities and the overproduction of doctors in America has led to the rise as patient as consumer. Again the British NHS has aped this system in recent years but with a centralised, budget controlled system it leaves the hospitals in the UK always overspent, trying to find ways of balancing their budgets. At least in the US if you attract more patients you get more money for the hospital. In the UK this has never quite been the case.

Even more than in the UK, the newspapers and the media in the States are full of medical stories which are often detailed and expertly written. The public is better informed and inherently curious and critical. Once in the city centre, I heard two middle-aged women debating the value of faecal occult blood testing as a screening tool for the diagnosis of colorectal cancer. Such a conversation would be rare at home even now.

Even on the wards the patients wanted information. Every fine detail of their surgery was explained. Every complication discussed. Every option outlined. This is desirable in many ways but its disadvantage is that it is very time-consuming.

I remember a ward round with the chief of surgery. A patient of thirty with worsening ulcerative colitis and in poor health who was finally going to need her colon removed and an ileo-anal pouch constructed in its place. All medical treatments had failed and she needed to be convinced of this. I watched as the surgeon over thirty minutes explained everything in great detail. Naturally there was plenty of emotion on display. The patient was from New York and a thousand miles from home. She had sought out the Cleveland Clinic because of its reputation.

'Now Mrs. Childs I hope I have explained it all fully. Is there any aspect you are not happy with?'

'Thank you doctor you have made it very clear but I would like you to talk to my gastroenterologist at home if you would.'

It was before the era of mobile phones but Mrs. Childs picked up the telephone by her bed and rang a New York number and handed the phone to the chief of surgery. It was her gastroenterologist. There then followed a twenty-five minute conversation between surgeon and physician on Mrs. Childs' behalf. I stood politely admiring the meticulous and unhurried way the consultation had been carried out. We had been standing by Mrs. Childs' bedside for more than fifty-five minutes and it was still not quite over.

Finally all parties were content and we moved on. There were twenty more patients to be seen before we could go home. No wonder the trainees never got home much before 10pm.

Mrs. Childs had her major operation the next day.

It was a success.

But I am not surprised that doctors, like most workers in the USA in those days thirty years ago, were only permitted to take two weeks holiday leave each year.

There were just not enough hours in the day or weeks in the year. Probably there still aren't.

***

It was George Bernard Shaw, the Irish playwright, who jested that England and America are two countries separated by the same language. My period in the US doing research certainly made me realise that this joke was more than accurate.

If Shaw had asked me I might have added that these two cultures were separated by a different sense of humour as well. My American friends certainly knew how to laugh and have fun over things that seemed rather fatuous to me but found my Englishman's ironic sense of humour difficult to respond to. I recall walking into a lift (elevator) and seeing a registrar (resident) I vaguely knew. He was wearing the loudest tie (necktie) I had ever seen. It was ghastly (gross).

I winked (flashed) knowingly and asked him who had vomited (puked) on his tie. In England I would have expected a laugh (chuckle) and then some sarcastic (snarky) quip in return. Instead my friend the resident nearly walloped (floored) me. Blimey (Jeez!) he really was angry (mad)!

From then on I was much more careful.

Noticing differences between English and the language used by Americans has a long tradition. Thomas Jefferson, the Virginian lawyer, who at the age of thirty-three was chiefly responsible for drafting the Declaration of Independence, was fascinated by words. He invented several. 'Belittle' was one of his neologisms that has stood the test of time on both sides of the Atlantic. Jefferson correctly wrote that judicious neology can give strength to language and enable it to be the vehicle of new ideas. Of course, changing language is another form of asserting difference and independence.

Far from being allergic to Americanisms I tried to understand them when in Ohio. 'You do the math' was amusing while 'touching base' irritating. Both phrases have become such clichés that they are almost unusable today. Worse of all is 'I dove' when the speaker should be saying 'I dived' into my research project. The lack of both the definite article and the preposition of a date, such as 'the operation took place 'first November' 1986', is ghastly.

One thing that has struck me in recent years since I returned from Cleveland is the foul language that Hollywood feeds us in bucket loads. It makes me eschew watching American cinema. Both the Californian lazy manner of speaking and the expletives make me want to switch off.

I never heard such language in Ohio or the eleven other states I visited in my time in the US. Everyone was generally very polite.

Except, of course, in New York.

**

There was only one thing missing for me during my time in Ohio. My new girl-friend Christina, the nursing sister, who I had dated the year before and would later marry. Towards the end of my time in Cleveland she flew over. It was the week before Christmas. There was three feet of snow in Shaker Heights with the snow ploughs starting work each morning at 4.30am. When she arrived I introduced her to my new-found friends and work colleagues and showed her Lake Erie and the cross-country skiing on the golf course near where I lived. A couple of days later we headed off on a grand tour of the country.

Purchasing a roving ticket with Delta Airlines allowed us to go anywhere anytime over a fortnight. We made use of this extraordinary deal and explored ten states. In Tennessee we stayed with a man who had founded a school. In Florida we sponged off an acquaintance in Fort Lauderdale and in Dallas we enjoyed the high rise city centre. In Arizona we marvelled at the Grand Canyon and in Los Angeles felt terribly threatened in the downtown area where it was clear drugs were being violently bought and sold in quantity. In San Francisco we enjoyed Chinatown and the Golden Gate Bridge and in Chicago, Illinois, downtown was as thrilling as people had said it was.

Everywhere we were made welcome. Being hospitable is the American way and we benefited greatly from this custom. Our British accents often stopped the crowds.

'Oh Gee! Can you say that again? Oh that's cute! I just love your accent.'

There was a child-like, almost naive quality in many of the people we met. We both admired, and were disturbed, by it. America is a country of extremes. High mountains, lakes and deserts. Urban sophisticates with encyclopaedic knowledge of the world and small town hillbillies who had never travelled from their town or even to the nearest city.

Such a land of contrasts.

But oddly, to my dismay, much of urban USA physically and culturally looked the same from one end to the other. Walking down a street in Florida did not feel much different than one in Arizona. The same big US-wide chains and franchises selling the same goods or peddling the same foods. For America's inhabitants it gave them a sense of being at home in any part of this vast continent thirty-five times bigger than my country. But for me coming from a continent such as Europe where the culture, history, language and architecture change radically every hundred miles there was a disappointing absence of variety. It was thus a great deal less fascinating.

Many years later I found the same monochrome culture was to be found in every part of the continent called Australia. Disappointing there too, though the geography of both continents is fascinating.

Christina's time in the US was short and we said goodbye knowing I had a month to finish up at the Cleveland Clinic before I would too be heading back to England. She had been impressed by America. Its optimism. Its energy. Its ambition. But like me she had no desire to stay. We loved our life at home and it would take more than a few skyscrapers overlooking Lake Michigan or the Everglades of Florida to change our plans.

As I typed up my research, publishing articles on the most appropriate diet for patients with Crohn's disease and our ability to predict recurrent disease patterns, I did not have any regrets. I was eager to resume my life in Britain. Although its murky weather, public reserve and self-deprecating people are somewhat wearying features at times, it was still my home.

And back home I would go.

Flaws and all, I could not wait to get back to continue my training in surgery in the United Kingdom.

Chapter 19: From Medical Student To Surgeon

❖

As I approach the end of my working life and the final glide to oblivion, I find myself wanting to lend a hand to those that are just starting out. Although I have enjoyed teaching medical students all my working life, I recently volunteered to become a tutor for the medical students at Imperial College London, to which Northwick Park Hospital is affiliated.

The system had been set up to guide the students as they negotiate the path through their medical studies. Sort of pastoral care and fatherly advice. Some students need help while others fly solo with confidence from an early age.

Reading my diaries from my time I am reminded as a medical student how strong and relatively sophisticated my opinions were at eighteen but also how muddled I was. I am sure the medical students of today are no different and benefit from a helping hand. Some will need much counselling. Others very little.

When I run my annual Open Day for School Students at Northwick Park my first question to the students is: 'What is the reason you are choosing medicine as a career?'

I receive a range of replies from those that are daring enough to hold up the microphone and contribute to the hundred others listening. The meeker ones stay silent.

'To help others.'

'Because I enjoy science.'

'To be respected.'

'To earn a good wage.'

Sadly and often from the first generation British whose families have fought hard to get to the UK: 'Because my parents want me to become a doctor.'

I then tell them that I was lucky to have decided to become a doctor at twelve years of age after watching Emergency Ward Ten, the precursor of Holby City and Casualty. I wanted to be one of those earnest doctors chatting over coffee as to how they might help their patients. Fantasy. Dreams. But life is nothing without them. My enthusiasm now at seventy is no different now than it was then. But as if to open their eyes to the danger of my idealism, I show them pictures of how unpleasant and unglamorous medicine, and, particularly, surgery can be. The sights, the smells, the misery and the sad times.

But then I tell them of the doctors that are coming to speak to them during the course of the day. I tell them that each one will use the F-word without my prompting. F for FUN. They will emphasise the hard work, the book learning and the long hours but all will conclude that it has been lots of FUN.

I remind them that doctors are privileged to treat fellow humans at their most vulnerable moments. We are trusted to look after their loved ones. We cannot sort out every problem but our job is to diagnose their ills, ease their pains and generally reduce their suffering.

What could be better than that?

And doctors are paid well enough.

Although doctors may not be the richest folk on Acacia Avenue, they are pretty close to the leafy end. This was illustrated clearly to me when, during my long search for advancement, I stopped at a garage in an attractive county town in the north of England to fill my car with fuel.

It had been a long journey and I got talking to the attendant.

'I am thinking of moving up here and, as house prices in the south where I come from are high, I might be able to afford a house in the nicer part of town. Where would that be exactly?'

Without knowing who or what I was the woman promptly replied:

'Oh, you mean where the doctors live?'

In my village in Hertfordshire those that live in the biggest houses are bankers and hedge fund managers who have large properties with lawns, gazebos and neat herbaceous borders. But they are troubled. Not only do they have to travel constantly in the course of their employment and may be away many nights of the year in some soulless hotel in a strange land, it seems that they are not quite happy in their work. Money they may have but, as time passes, they learn that is only a small part of the story of a happy life. Working for organisations that only think of money as their goal is deeply unsatisfactory. Some retire early to play endless rounds of golf while others become teachers in their fifties.

I remind the students that it is job satisfaction and life-time fulfilment that are the most important features of any career. Now that we are in Covid-19 times another vital strength of medical work is that we are recession proof.

My next question to these young men and women is:

'Are you planning, or have had, gap years?'

The majority answer is a depressing NO!

I then illustrate my depth of feeling about the need to get out of the academic factory of medicine and into the outside world as often as possible. I illustrate this with my own experience.

I left school at seventeen with the qualifications needed for medicine and headed for a mission hospital in Africa. Working there and travelling around in Zululand was a formative experience and I started at University College London the next year refreshed. This experience expanded my horizons and, although I was the same age as my peers on that first day at medical school, I had gleaned a slight sophistication that they may have lacked.

For two years I worked hard dissecting bodies and performing physiology experiments but found I needed to escape again. Luckily I had been the president of the Medical Society so that when I came to asking the impossible question 'Can you keep my place open for me so I might work abroad for a while?' My request may have received horrified looks but the door was not slammed in my face and they let me go.

'We will not see you again probably?' the dean had said.

He was wrong, for after an overland trek across Asia and nine months working in Indian hospitals, I was back ready to continue.

I am convinced that times away from the core activity of a career develops the individual much beyond the time taken up by that adventure. After all we are training these doctors for fifty-year careers so what is the rush? Moreover I have noticed that I am quizzed more in medical interviews about those times away than I am about my formal research efforts or clinical activity in my chosen field. It seems that even the stay-at-homes admire the go-getters who expand their minds by expanding their experiences.

I am not sure my arguments convince my students.

'But I don't want to miss the opportunities when they come.'

'But I will never be able to pay back my student loans if I go away.'

'My parents would not countenance such a plan.'

I listen to these arguments unimpressed.

One day they will look back and learn that they were wrong and I was right.

***

Recalling my days as a medical student after fifty years is a nostalgic, bitter-sweet affair. The cold lodgings and the lack of money. I could buy nothing more than the basics though the student union beer always seemed affordable. The shared cadaver to dissect. The early morning lectures on physical anthropology and biochemistry. The dark winter evenings and the hours in the library at University College Hospital.

But there was much to enjoy as well. I experimented with relationships. I directed plays and began to write. The rote learning of medicine did not quite offer enough creativity for me and I needed to escape into the arts. The huge effort of learning volumes of scientific fact-after-fact was wearying and tedious. Of course, like a language you need the grammar and vocabulary before you can converse. I was learning that language but it was hard.

I read once that mastering medicine demands a new supplementary vocabulary of 35,000 words. In a survey of 50,000 biomedical terms it was found that 58% were derived from Greek alone, 22% from Latin alone, 13% oddly combine Greek and Latin and only 3% originate from English or a modern language.

That sounds daunting to medical students but I remind them that, even if they have never studied Greek and Latin, they know advanced English. All our complex words are made up of Greek or Latin anyway. This means they know already what the prefixes and suffixes in any medical term mean.

When I say this they look at me blankly so I illustrate it with an example: 'If I use the word metachronous in relation to a colon cancer you can tell me after a little thought what it means?'

That stumps most of them but after a moment a bright spark asks:

'Doesn't chronos mean time in Ancient Greek?'

'Yes, well done, hence the word in medicine 'chronic' to express an illness over time. If you had a watch on your arm you might call it by the fancier name 'chronometer', a measure of time. So what is metachronous? Think about another word that includes meta. Like metamorphosis.'

'Does meta mean change?'

'Exactly it is a Greek preposition used as a prefix meaning among, between, or by way of change. Metamorphosis means changing shape. So back to metachronous?'

'A change in time perhaps?' Another bright one adds.

'Right! A second tumour which appears in the colon at a different time is a metachronous one. It occurs in 5% of colon cancers suggesting that surveillance after a cancer operation would be a good thing.'

My tortuous attempts at getting the students to think about the language of medicine continues.

'The rectum is named because it is a straight part of the colon (see rectangular – Latin rectus straight and angulus angle) and diagnosis means 'through knowledge' (Greek dia through and gnōsis knowledge)…'

I look around the seminar room and half the students have their eyes shut tight. Are they thinking hard or just trying to sleep through my lecture?

I hope one or two at least have had their eyes opened etymologically?

I am not sure.

**

When I returned from India after that second gap year I began to walk the wards and clerk patients. It was then the excitement of medicine as a grown-up career began to grow. There was the uniform. I wore a short white coat in those days to be distinguished from the qualified staff who wore long white ones. I would ask patients every question I could think of that was relevant to them. I would write these down on index cards and tick them off. The process would take hours and the patients often got bored though most loved the attention I was giving them. An old man with urinary problems would be asked about: haematuria (blood), nocturia (night-time), dysuria (pain), oliguria (little), polyuria (lots), pollakiuria (frequent), etc.

It would all take quite a lot of interpretation but little by little I became more fluent.

University College Hospital conducted impressive medical meetings where the great physicians of the hospital would pontificate at Grand Rounds. These events were conducted almost like gladiatorial fights with the registrars presenting complex cases which the professors and senior consultants would pick apart. They would fight like tigers for a particular piece of the story that they could make their own.

Often the patient was present and would end up being labelled with the most extraordinarily rare, esoteric diagnosis. In the days before good imaging a lot of these diagnoses were highly speculative. They could neither be proved nor disproved. The more obscure the condition the cleverer must be the doctor who suggested it. Sometimes the outcome of these discussions would seem to be pure fancy.

After an exhausting hour or two in the Grand Round we students would head to the postmortem room before lunch and watch the latest dead body being dissected and analysed. These were always great teaching sessions for the answer to the patient's illness was usually apparent. With cupped hands the morbid pathologist would hold up the liver and demonstrate the extent of the cirrhosis or show us a tumour in the colon. At other times they would slice through the brain with a huge knife and show us those confusing grey and white areas that we had been trying to understand with our own brains during those long hours in the library.

These autopsy (Greek autos = self and opsis = view) events were so impressive that, when I was a houseman and trying to decide what specialty to follow, I conducted a few postmortems under supervision. It was fascinating work but I decided definitively that I would rather spend a lifetime holding warm, living organs in my hands than putting them in perishingly (Latin perire = to pass away entirely) cold bodies.

Whoops, sorry! No more etymological torture.

I promise that will be the last Latin and Greek lesson.

***

In the popular public mind a surgeon is a doctor who is happiest when his patient is lifeless and asleep. A surgeon is a technician. Almost a geek if not a nerd. Surely they cannot be empathetic souls? Nowadays we are taught to avoid stereotypes and I think this one is about as bad as stereotypes can be.

I chose surgery as a career because it can change lives so dramatically. The results are often immediate. But it was a close call. As a student I was very interested in psychiatry. UCH excelled at this. I had read much Freud, Jung, and Adler and the Department of Psychiatry offered volunteer students to take on their own patients for long-term psychotherapy sessions.

Every week for a year I would see my patient, who had been selected as suitable by Dr. Wolff, the consultant psychiatrist. He would supervise half a dozen students together each week. I would describe the conversations with my patient, who was a neurotic women of about my own age, and be given guidance as to how to conduct the sessions to come. It was an invaluable and most rewarding exercise but came to an end after two years when I qualified after counselling my second patient, a young man, a flasher of his genitals, who kept exposing himself on the underground train near Piccadilly Circus.

This exposure to psychotherapy was a major influence in my medical training and I still use some of the lessons I learnt then in my day to day approach to my surgical patients.

Many of the best times being at UCH as a student were the periods when I was not actually there. The first of these away months was in an asylum in Denbigh, North Wales. One of the psychiatrists linked to UCH practised widely in Wales. He invited us to fly up to Denbigh in his little plane from Biggin Hill Aerodrome in Kent. Did all consultants earn so much that they could afford their own aeroplane? We were impressed but he was an exception as I learnt later he had the largest private practice in the principality.

That month in north Wales showed me the other half of the psychiatric coin. Locked away for years in the asylum were many who today are in sheltered accommodation in the community or sleeping rough on our streets. I studied in three asylums during the course of my training and, although I did not find the atmosphere cruel, the modern way is probably better.

In my fourth year I learnt how to deliver babies and after a good grounding at UCH, I found myself in Bedford General Hospital locked away for a month on the labour ward. With a good friend who was seconded with me, together we delivered every available baby in Bedfordshire. It was exhilarating but exhausting but I was so enthused that I went in for the Obstetric Essay prize and won a scholarship.

A month living in the home of a GP in Hebden Bridge, Yorkshire gave me the idea that life as a GP would be quite attractive. The independence of running your own practice forging it in your own way seemed very appealing. Unfortunately this dream of autonomy for GPs in the NHS has been soured by this independence being overridden by prescriptive directives from their paymaster, the government. GPs in Britain are self-employed partnerships mostly but now have the unenviable position of being treated as an employee but having none of the direct benefits of being one. What was once a very attractive field now struggles to recruit and retain its doctors.

I admired the family doctor, cradle-to-grave concept of general practice, but in the end it was the jack-of-all-trades-master-of-none ethos of general practice that finally pushed me to become a specialist. I would become a doctor who would finally know everything about nothing, as the saying goes.

Students spend a lot of time dreaming of their elective period, where they choose anywhere in the world to study for three or four months. I decided to learn Spanish by spending my summer with a family in Madrid. Then I headed for small town Venezuela. In those more stable days for that oil-rich country the hospital in Guiria within sight of the island of Trinidad was a sleepy well-appointed place. I worked in the laboratory and on the wards and enjoyed the beach and the amistad of my Venezuelan co-workers.

No-one in the town spoke a word of English so unwittingly I became an interpreter for the many Trinidadian fishermen who the Venezuelan coastguard took great delight in throwing into prison whenever they came a metre into their territorial waters. Visiting them in the police cells where they appeared badly treated was a sobering experience.

A stint at the Tropical Medicine School in Caracas gave me a good grounding in parasitology and helped me understand a lot more of the parasites I had seen down the microscope in Guiria. Back in England our patients are lucky to have so few of these irritating organisms in their guts to compete with.

But the most significant month away from UCH, and one which would change the direction of my life, was in a town in north Hampshire with a swanky new hospital. Basingstoke does not have a particularly magical ring to it. Perhaps as a new town it has too many roundabouts and a skyscraper plonked right in the middle. Perhaps the name is just inelegant? I am not sure why it should always raise a wry smile. This reputation is not deserved.

The new hospital was built in the grounds of Park Prewitt Mental Hospital and was well designed. It attracted high calibre consultants from London who pulled in plenty of patients from the surrounding countryside. Many of these consultants were keen to initiate research projects as well.

When I arrived there in 1974 as a student in surgery it was already busy. From the start I felt involved in a way I had not been at UCH where there had been too many students to compete with. At Basingstoke I worked all hours with the result that even as a fourth year student I was able to perform two supervised appendicectomies. It was exhilarating. This was good work. Here I sensed the thrill that I was making an immediate difference to a patient's health.

The consultants were active and keen. A new consultant Bill Heald exuded an enthusiasm I had rarely encountered before. Indirectly he would change the direction of my life. All trainees follow by example. Heald was passionate about his work particularly in the field of rectal cancer where he would go on to make a major international contribution. I felt pulled along after him in his slipstream.

So it was into the discipline of general surgery I would go.

Benefitting from my experiences away from the teaching hospital at UCH, I had seen how medicine could be practised in the district hospital setting. Without the distraction and bitter rivalries of university departments and their ambitious professors.

A surgeon I would become.

I knew then it would be to the district general hospitals I would go to gain the experience I needed.

**

I qualified in June 1975, and after a few locums I began work as a house physician for a cardiologist in that very same hospital in Basingstoke.

My career as a doctor had finally started. It was long hours of hard work but I loved every minute of it. I mastered caring for strokes, heart attacks, pneumonia and patients in diabetic coma. I even published a paper entitled Psittacosis myocarditis describing the first case in the world of pigeon fancier's bad heart.

As a houseman I was on duty every other night and weekend in addition to working full days. On duty I slept in the doctor's room attached to the ward. It was pleasant enough and fairly clean. I got a few hours' sleep each night as I was often being called to the wards to put in intravenous lines or urinary catheters. I did not sleep well in my small room but it was a welcome refuge. One that got me through the long nights ready for the working day ahead.

One evening I was called to attend to an old man in heart failure brought on by his longstanding aortic valve disease. Left ventricular failure is characterised by breathlessness, cough and crepitations, or crackles, at the base of the lungs when listening with a stethoscope. His heart was irregular and I made an additional diagnosis of atrial fibrillation. The gentleman was cyanosed and puffing away. He was near to drowning because of the fluid that had accumulated in his lungs. A chest X-ray and an electrocardiogram quickly confirmed my findings. I administered both digitalis by mouth and a strong diuretic, frusemide, intravenously.

As if by magic over the next ten minutes he came back to life and started talking. With oxygen at maximum strength his colour improved and I noted his urinary catheter was draining urine at a great rate into the bag attached to the bed. Within twenty minutes he was asking for a cup of tea and a biscuit. With the patient out of danger I could get back to my little room.

It was five o'clock in the morning and I wanted to get some sleep before the day began.

As I walked along the corridor I noticed I must have left the door of my room opened. Careless of me. No matter though because there was not much money in my jacket and it was in the days before credit cards. The light was off and I fell into the bed ready to sleep for as long as I could.

I suddenly realised I was not alone.

I felt an arm on my shoulder and heard some light breathing.

Worse than that the bed was decidedly wet.

Minnie, aged 87, was quietly lying next to me in my bed.

I knew Minnie quite well. I had treated her on the adjoining ward for a mild stroke and dementia and she was due to get home in a day or two.

Unfortunately although she was normally fairly continent of urine she had made an exception once tucked up in the warmth of my bed. I jumped out and called her ward.

After the patient had been escorted back and the bed changed I lost my desire for sleep.

I headed for the canteen to be first in for breakfast at 6.30am.

***

It was the mother of a now famous TV personality who asked me a telling question after a long weekend looking after her. She was dying from primary biliary cirrhosis. Her liver damaged beyond hope. I expect today she might be a candidate for a liver transplant but then it was an experimental treatment only.

I had seen her many times over the weekend as she needed lines changed, drug doses altered and much besides. I was in and out morning, noon and certainly night. She was always brave, charming and cheerful despite her plight. I had plenty of time for her as she had known my mother when they were in the WRENs together during the war and they were still vaguely in touch.

'Do you resent giving up your young life in the hospital, Peter? You have been here all weekend day and night and I know you are on duty this coming week as well. How do you do it and why?'

The question stopped me in my tracks for a moment. It was a good question but I already knew what my response would be.

'No, not really! It is a privilege to treat people like you, Jane. It is not a burden. It is a privilege.'

With that I rushed off to see another patient.

I cannot exactly recall when Jane died but I do not think it was very long after this conversation.

I was sad, of course.

But a doctor cannot mourn long for his patients. There are always plenty more Janes waiting for attention in our hospitals. Morning, noon and night.

Chapter 20:
Medicine, Music And Laughter

❖

Thinking of Jane's question makes me realise how several aspects of life can underpin the main aim. Obviously the support of family and friends are central but for me too music and laughter have sustained me in this life of service to my patients.

I am sure this would be the same in many other professions.

***

Music and medicine seem to mesh well.

Laughter is an incongruous bedfellow.

The learning of music by rote and then the expressing of it with emotion and originality mirrors the same process that I went through at medical school, learning the grammar and vocabulary of medicine. I had to learn the language before I could dance within its boundaries. This process was arduous and occasionally joyless, as I have indicated. Sometimes I thought my head would burst with the volume of stuff that had to be learnt. But little by little the constant, repetitive routines led to a kind of cognitive medical intelligence.

One day came a revelation. As with any new language I began to dream in it. Those strange half-Greek, half-Latin medical words that thousands of doctors had fabricated in the seventeenth and eighteenth centuries became second nature to me. Without knowing exactly when I, not quite an MBBS let alone an FRCS, was grasped by the growing gift of medical fluency. Perhaps others are asked to balance on the head of a pin, but I, and my medical school chums, had learnt to pirouette in the dialect of semiology, the signs and symptoms of disease.

It had been a moment when the fascination of medicine had first been unveiled and the miracle of it has never left me. I remember a brilliant professor saying on the radio once that medicine and surgery were a very straightforward subject that could easily be mastered. I have never found that to be the case at all. Perhaps I do not have the intellect, and maybe that's not a bad thing. If you have too much intellect you will probably not be a good physician or surgeon. You might be a good researcher but not a good doctor, looking after the mundane aspects of patient care as well as the more challenging problems.

Whatever the truth, I am sure the professor was actually wrong. Medicine is a vast landscape of uncertainty and complexity which might take more than a dozen medical lifetimes to truly master.

I doubt anyone, anywhere has ever done so.

I certainly have not.

***

These parallels with music might explain why many doctors are quite good musicians. The fact that it is good to have hobbies outside medicine to take your mind off the stresses of the day job is another consideration. In my case I began to learn music seriously as a teenager, which meant I could never be much good. A virtuoso must begin to play as a toddler.

That last sentence is interesting when we consider the fact that we do not teach the technical side of surgery and medicine until doctors are in their late twenties. None of us would ever pay money to see a musician who started playing at that late stage of development. Yet our patients put themselves in the hands of surgeons who do not really start honing their skills much before they are twenty-five.

Back to music.

My identical twin and I led the orchestra at school as duplicate lead violinists. One term he would lead and the next I would. Being identical no-one ever knew the difference between us so it all worked out perfectly. Music was a good way to get through the stresses of the teenage years but it was a decade later before I took music up again.

I had rebelled against the staid, middle-class aura of the classical music setting. The audiences were quiet, polite and well-dressed. They never hollered or stood on their chairs in ecstasy. I am sure they enjoyed themselves hugely but I was looking for something a lot more demonstrative.

I began playing rock music. Guitar, harmonica and rock fiddle but found the musicians I played with used the volume of their amplifiers as their main musical expression. They did not listen to each other much but just played louder until the sound became a cacophony. Escaping from this noise it was logical that I moved into folk music, fiddle in hand. I founded a band with a banjo/bazooki player named David and we began to rehearse. A year later we were a seven piece traditional folk group called Innominata. A name I made up as I could not think of a decent one.

We began to play out and were paid modestly for our efforts. Three albums, two small British tours and two hundred and fifty gigs followed over the next decade. It was a great escape from medicine. I learnt a lot about performance and audiences. I learnt that an audience, like those classical ones in the hallowed concert halls, may indeed enjoy themselves hugely without the need to be standing on their seats yelling. I also learnt that a small audience could enjoy themselves as much as, if not more than, a larger one.

These lessons were useful in my medical career later when I began to lecture to students and others.

After a decade of playing imitation Celtic folk music I was forced to give up Innominata when I relocated to Northwick Park Hospital ninety miles to the north. It was just too far away to be an active band member.

I regret hugely this and although I have played music sporadically with others since I have never been able to reproduce the family feeling and shared ambition that Innominata afforded me. I am pleased to know that they are still playing regularly but glad to know that their founder front man's disappearance is still mourned a little.

***

Finding myself at Northwick Park with the responsibilities of a growing family and a demanding job, I needed an outlet for this the showy side of my character. What could I do to get me in front of an audience but not depend on others? Most of my colleagues seemed satisfied with the buzz of medical conferences with their plenary session audiences and sharp question and answer exchanges from fellow doctors.

Somehow surgical conferences never appealed to me greatly and year-on-year they became shockingly repetitious. The same clever doctors showing off their research findings in front of the same other doctors year on year. Somehow it did not float my boat. Perhaps that was because I knew I could not compete with them as my research efforts, data collection, delegation skills and eye for detail have always been only modest.

No, it would have to be something else.

It was about that time I was asked to do an after-dinner speech to the local Rotary Club in Harrow. I prepared hard and it went well. Suddenly I realised I had a new skill to learn but, if I was lucky, the audiences would be so well fastened to their seats after their main course that they would not have the temerity to escape until after I had completed my task. One of the principles I later learnt which gave the speaker a competitive advantage was that the speaker should be stone cold sober and the audience tipsy.

It was time to write some original material. My aim was to illustrate the serious and non-serious side of being a surgeon. My purpose would be to educate and amuse in equal measure. At first I called it Giblets and Tripe but in later years I have called it Stupidity and Redemption as I contrast the madness of the administrative system I work in with the courage and humour of the patients I am fortunate to serve.

I began writing and collecting suitable material and signed up with a few professional speaking agencies.

And so another little adventure began.

Emphasising the witty side of surgery was not illogical as I have observed over many years just how important humour and laughter is to the practice of medicine. Even when patients are experiencing their darkest moments of pain, fear and uncertainty, it was so often their humour and wit which brought them out of these miserable corners of despair. I have learnt to support them with humour and with a wink and a smile. It is a technique to be used carefully, always trying to find the most appropriate moment to lighten the patients' load.

It mostly works.

As laughter has been said to be the best medicine, there was plenty of material to access in joke books. Most of it was banal rubbish. Only occasionally would I stumble across a story or a joke I could use. But, if I heard anyone else using it, I would never employ it again. It is odd that humour must always appear new and original while music in the form of songs at a live rock concert, for example, is best appreciated when the audience has heard them fifty times before and can sing along. That is one of the reasons I consider it must be much harder to be a good comedian than a rock star. Perhaps that is why most comedians do not come to prominence until they are in their thirties.

I worked hard collecting suitable material that fitted in with the medical stories I was trying to tell. I filled a box with thousands of jokes and pored over them whenever I prepared a talk.

Better still was to write my own material. There was plenty to write about. I had observed the problem that patients have with doctors and their titles. Dr., Mr., Miss, Mrs., Ms., Professor, etc. and the odd way that the medical profession did everything it could to confuse the patient more. As I thought about it I realised my own title had changed five times in my life.

It made a perfect palindrome.

When I was a little boy I suppose I was a 'master'.

But then I reached eighteen and the age of consent and so became a 'mister'.

After five years at medical school I qualified and so became a 'doctor'.

But having decided to become a surgeon I studied for the Diploma of the Royal College of Surgeons of England and five years later again became a 'mister'.

But to become a consultant in the NHS I was forced to do a higher degree after some two years of full-time research I achieved a Mastership in Surgery. So I became a 'master' again!

From master to mister to doctor to mister to master!

Seems like it was a lot of work for nothing! Reminds me of the ditty:

There was a young man called Breeze
Weighed down with MAs and MDs
He collapsed from the strain
Said his doctor 'it's plain
You are killing yourself with degrees!'

This usually made the crowd chuckle but when I got on the subject of my particular profession of coloproctology they squirmed and laughed in equal measure. I often took them by surprise when I told them that:

I was a bowel surgeon interested in taking out tripes, lights, sweet breads, gall-bladders and the occasional onion. But that my real interest is, or rather are, HAEMORRHOIDS. At that point, I would wonder why there was a ripple of awkward laughter going round the room as I knew that at least half of them were sitting on their haemorrhoids at the present time.

After all, I reminded them, it is said there are two kinds of people in the world. Those that admit to haemorrhoids and liars. They are incredibly common.

I would then regale my audience with the history of my subject. From the Pharaoh Senruset in Upper Egypt who had a courtier known as the Shepherd-of-the-Royal-Anus to Louis XIV, le roi soleil, whose three fistula-in-ano procedures made his brave surgeon Dr. Felix one of the richest doctors in Europe.

With jokes about being a proctologist wanting always to have a job where I could feel the wind in my hair or with Henry Ford's quip that the problem with the human body is that the exhaust is too near the ignition, I amused the diners. My supplementary aim was to give them a taste of surgery so I take them through an appendicectomy with its descriptive language and smells.

Sometimes the least subtle jokes seemed to be received the best. That is the mystery of audiences. Here's one.

In the history of coloproctology, which I cover in detail, I also mention an Ionian Greek doctor called Soranus who was really a gynaecologist. This unsubtle line always brings the house down. Don't ask me why but I won't drop it while it stills gets that laugh.

It was all good clean (?) fun and I have dined out on my material a couple of hundred times. But it was the stories of patients and what they have said to me which intrigued my listeners more. They are the redemption while the politics of medicine is the stupidity.

An example:

Once, when I was performing a sigmoidoscopy for rectal bleeding on a young British Airways hostess to make sure she did not have colitis, she looked over her shoulder and demanded brashly:

'Has anyone ever done this to you, Mr. McDonald? Huh! Do you know what it feels like?'

I thought for a moment, thinking of her job on the aeroplanes, before replying.

'Young lady, before they allow you to serve your customers, do they make you experience a crash a few times?'

I think that kept her quiet.

Things patients say to me are so illuminating and are so extraordinarily illogical at times that they make me chuckle quietly. I remember having to tell a fifty-five year old woman who had presented with back pain that her scan had unfortunately shown a cancer of the pancreas. A diagnosis always fatal, I was expecting a difficult reaction.

Instead she said: 'Oh well, Mr. McDonald, at least it's not gall-stones!'

This time it was me who was quiet for a minute or two.

A true story I tell in my routine was of the urology registrar at Basingstoke Hospital who was so tired he fell asleep when doing a rectal examination. The poor fellow had been up all weekend and the room was poorly ventilated.

Another story, that was not true, was how the patient had demanded a double digit examination on his prostate so he could get an immediate second opinion.

I would recall an actual consultation I had with an old man in 1983. It was at the height of the newly recognised HIV epidemic. Most doctors then were as ignorant of the details of this terrible slow virus as the general public. We were learning fast and, for the first time in our careers, had all been urged routinely to take a sexual practice history. It was really rather embarrassing as we were unused to this but we knew we had to bite the bullet. I plucked up enough courage and began:

'I am sorry Mr. White but I am obliged to ask you nowadays because of the recent problem of AIDS if you are homosexual or heterosexual?'

I articulated the words clearly and rather slowly to give Mr. White, who was rather deaf, time to think.

A few moments later he replied:

'Homosexual? Heterosexual? Mr. McDonald. They're all perverts!'

Needless to say, I did not frame the question quite the same way from that day on.

Slowly I learnt more of the tricks of the speaking trade. I noticed several things about after-dinner audiences. The first was that all-male audiences were harder to warm up than mixed ones. The ladies seemed to laugh louder and more spontaneously than the men. If it was a mixed audience, the men would follow the ladies' example and let their hair down. The best audience was an all-female crowd. I once spoke to two hundred freemason's wives at their annual dinner. They nearly lifted off the roof with their laughter. Maybe there was a touch of a hen's night hysteria that evening that made my job easy. It was memorable.

The second lesson I learnt was never to get on your feet too late. As the evening wears on and the auxiliary speakers ramble on and on, boring their audiences with awards and badly prepared stories, many of the diners fall asleep. Many cannot wait to go home or get to the bar to escape the tedium. This underlined to me the principle that the audience should be both tipsy and awake for the show to be a success. So much so that I tell organisers that I will not start speaking after 10pm.

This point is so important that frequently I use a borrowed story.

The president of a society was waiting patiently to introduce their guest after-dinner speaker. But last year's president was drivelling on about his time in office. It was very, very boring. Finally, the new president could wait no longer. In a pique of anger, he picked up the heavy wooden gavel in front of him and banged it on the table. Unfortunately, in doing so he let the gavel slip out of his hand and it hit his neighbour, the after dinner speaker, very hard on the forehead. So much so that he slid under the table in a semi-conscious state.

As the esteemed guest's head disappeared under the level of the tablecloth the president heard him say.

'For God's sake! Please, Mr. President, hit me again. This time harder. I can still hear the bugger!'

I lambast the politicians and the managers and their management-speak communiqués. I make fun of the earnest courses they make us all do to fulfil health and safety requirements. I remind my audience that management is often about being seen to do something rather than necessarily achieving it.

Much of this activity just produces chaos and confusion rather than enlightenment.

The surgeon, the architect and the politician are arguing that each of their professions is the oldest.
The surgeon begins.
'Well, we took a rib from Adam and we made Eve!'
'Surgery must be the oldest profession.'
'Nonsense!' retorts the architect.
'After all, we took all of the chaos and built the world. Yes! We took all that chaos and built the world!'
'Architecture must be the oldest profession.'
The politician looked at them both disdainfully.
'No you're both wrong! Politics is the oldest profession because who do you think created all the chaos in the first place!'

***

When they have had plenty I finish with the following poem that was written by that prolific writer Anon but adapted by me:

The old surgeon stood at the Heavenly Gate
His face was lined and old.
He stood before the man of Fate
For admission to the fold.

'What have you done?' Saint Peter said
'To gain admission here?'
'I've worked for the National Health Service, Sir
For many and many a year.'

The Pearly Gate swung open wide
As Saint Peter touched the bell
'Come in and take a harp, my dear,
You've had your share of Hell!'

Of course, this is not quite my true sentiment.

As I have hinted in this memoir elsewhere, there are many flaws with the nationalised, monolithic, planned, top-down NHS. But, it might be, just as Winston Churchill said of democracy in 1947, that the NHS is a bad health system but that the others are worse still. Some problems would disappear if it was restructured. Other problems would be exacerbated. New difficulties and inequalities would appear. A better system would certainly be costlier and improvements do not always last.

It may be that the NHS is the best of many bad alternative structures when viewed from all interested parties. If that is the case we need to state it regularly but we should worry that no debate about how we fund the NHS is now possible. Since the NHS was formed in 1948, politicians of all hues in the UK have hardly dared to speak of reforming its principles. As a concept it is frozen, petrified, unquestioned. That is not a healthy position for a health system to be in.

It is not for want of trying to improve it but without tackling the conundrum of how it is funded, we are frozen in time. It is said that in Britain we do not have social revolutions, just re-organisations of the NHS. In my lifetime in the NHS I have lived through half a dozen major reforms. Not one of these has been a success. Most have just fizzled out. Sometimes we find ourselves back where we were decades before.

A merry-go-round that keeps revolving.

***

The Plan

In the beginning was The Plan
And then came The Assumptions
And The Assumptions were without Form
And The Form was completely without Substance

And darkness fell upon the face of the Health Workers
And they sayeth unto their Clinical Directors
'It is a crock of shit and it stinketh!'

And the Clinical Directors
Went unto the Chief Executives
And sayeth unto them
'It is a vessel of fertiliser
And none may abide its stench!'

And the Chief Executives went nigh unto the Secretary of State for Health
And sayeth unto Him
'This Plan seems very strong and rather powerful!'

And the Secretary of State went to the Prime Minister

And sayeth unto Him
'This powerful new Plan will promote growth and efficiency in the Health Service as we know it!'

And the Prime Minister looked upon The Plan
And thought that it was good.
And from that day henceforth
It became yet another New NHS Plan.

Amen.
(Anon)

***

In the meantime, if we want our patients to smile when they go home, let us, perhaps, give them a free prescription of music and laughter on discharge just to make sure.

Chapter 21:
Did He Save Lives?

❖

My work in defence of doctors that I related in Chapter 4 provides a backdrop for an event that happened in the private hospital just a mile from Northwick Park Hospital.

Let me tell you a tragic tale.

***

David Sellu FRCS was a consultant surgeon in the NHS. His main base was Ealing General Hospital in West London. He had been born in Sierra Leone in either 1948 or 1950. Neither he nor his parents, who were subsistence farmers, could quite remember. David was the eldest of ten children and for the first twelve years of his life he wore no shoes and lived in a house without running water.

David was very bright and was given an opportunity to go to a good school where he studied hard. He eventually passed his Cambridge external examinations and miraculously won a place to study medicine at Manchester University. Qualifying six years later he went on to train as a surgeon and became a Fellow of two Royal Colleges of Surgeons.

After a five year stint as a consultant helping to set up a medical school in Oman, he was appointed a consultant general surgeon with an interest in colorectal surgery at both the Hammersmith and Ealing hospitals in West London. By then, he was married and embarking on a family with his wife Catherine, who would bear him four children.

He began practising privately at the Clementine Churchill Hospital in Harrow-on-the-Hill as well as keeping his NHS appointment. Being kind, calm and exceptionally hard-working, it was not long before his practice was flourishing. He overworked both in the public as well as the private sector and the rewards came in the form of good fees and hundreds of patients who adored him. Many were so grateful for his ministrations that they gave him many gifts in their appreciation of his care.

I first made David's acquaintance when he called me into theatre in the Clementine Churchill Hospital urgently to give a second opinion. On the operating table was a woman of forty-five with a cancer of the colon. Nothing particularly unusual about that but in those days before routine staging CT scans it was possible to be wrong-footed during an operation.

On performing the laparotomy, the incision in the belly, David had been horrified to find widespread peritoneal tumour which had spread throughout the abdominal cavity. This had not been anticipated. Hence the second opinion for reassurance and guidance.

As I looked on, I could see the tumour had invaded the both the lymph nodes near the colon, the liver itself, and the fat pad that hangs from the colon, the omentum. It was also caked with tumour. The cancer was everywhere inside the abdominal cavity and quite incurable.

'Thanks Peter for coming in to advise. I expect at St. Mark's Hospital you see plenty like this?'

'Certainly, David. Poor woman. All you can do is complete the primary resection of the right colon, take out as much of the omentum as you can and start chemotherapy when she has recovered.'

'Will do. Always a bit of shock when we get a nasty surprise, isn't it?'

'Indeed it is. Anyway, see you around David.'

This story illustrates clearly the surgeon that David Sellu had become. Cautious, caring and willing to ask for others' opinion and advice.

My portrait of this London surgeon originally from West Africa makes the story I am about to tell even more shocking.

***

It was 7.30pm on the evening of the 11th of February 2010, when David Sellu was in the middle of his private clinic at the Clementine Churchill Hospital. An operating day at Ealing Hospital had finished at 5pm before he had motored along the A40 to Harrow-on-the-Hill.

The telephone in his consulting room rang.

'Hello, Mr. Sellu? It's Mr. Hollingdale, the orthopaedic surgeon here. I think we may have met once or twice at meetings?'

'Ah yes. John isn't it?'

'That's right. I would be most grateful to have your advice about a patient in Blenheim Suite. A man I operated upon at the weekend. A total knee replacement which went without incident although I have put him on some antibiotics. But he has quite severe abdominal pain. Could you come and see, tonight?'

'Of course. I will pop in on my way home.'

The patient, Mr. Hughes, turned out to be sixty-six years old and was in some pain in the lower abdomen. David Sellu chatted to him and examined his tummy. His abdomen was quite tender and he was in pain. But he looked a good colour. Sellu checked his blood tests results and his X-rays.

'Mr. Hughes, I think it could be a puncture in part of your bowel after all those pain-killers you have had for your knee but I think a scan would be a good idea. I will get it as soon as possible. A change of antibiotics and some blood tests might be in order too. I'll pop in to see you again in the morning.'

Before he left the ward, Sellu had spoken on the telephone to the Resident Medical Officer about these changes. He got home to Hillingdon and ate a snack. He slept almost immediately his head touched the pillow.

At about 6.30am, Sellu received a call from the nurse on the ward telling him that Mr. Hughes' urine output had reduced. More intravenous fluids were prescribed and the urine flow picked up. Other than that the patient's condition was unchanged.

David skimmed in and out of Blenheim Ward at about 9.30am before starting an endoscopy list. Mr. Hughes looked much as he had the previous night. David noted the CT had still not been performed. He did not notice that there had been not been any changes made to the prescribed antibiotics. He was pleased that the intravenous fluids were continuing. At about midday David got a call from consultant radiologist Robin Kantor telling him the result of the scan.

'I think Mr. Hughes has a perforation of his sigmoid colon, David. Probably diverticular disease as there are some diverticula close by in the adjacent colon.'

Sellu had considered diverticular perforation a possible diagnosis. Pockets form in the colon with age and can get inflamed and perforate at any time. There is often not much warning when it happens. Especially if constipation is a complicating feature. From the tone of Robin Kantor's call, it was clear that the patient would need an operation, and soon.

David made a few phone calls but found that there was no theatre available that afternoon. Perhaps, he could get started at 5pm but he had to find an anaesthetist. The theatre staff did not have a rota of anaesthetists available despite the managers of the Clementine Churchill Hospital having been urged previously on more than one occasion to put one in place.

He began to call around his anaesthetic colleagues and many other anaesthetists who were not known to him. Apparently no-one was available. Finally, he found one who was anaesthetising for another surgeon that same afternoon at the Clementine Churchill. He would be available later at about 6pm. David went up at 4pm to Mr. Hughes to consent the patient. He noted that Mr. Hughes was now not feeling so well, but he was clinically stable. He could only wait and get into theatre as soon as possible.

It was after 5pm before Sellu's own list of colonoscopies was over. He still had not heard that theatre had sent for his patient. An hour later Mr. Hughes had still not been called for. The anaesthetist phoned him and told him of the delay.

'Mr. Sellu, I am afraid the gynaecology patient I am anaesthetising is in trouble, and we are calling out another surgeon urgently. It will be some time before we can operate on Mr. Hughes.'

Minutes became an hour. One hour became several. Sellu was patient but deeply frustrated. It was 10pm before they called for Mr. Hughes. As the patient was being anaesthetised and prepped for surgery, his blood pressure collapsed and extra intravenous lines had to be inserted. The intensivist from the ICU came to help. Finally, the operation got underway at about 11pm. A midline incision revealed faecal peritonitis from a perforated diverticulum and, unexpectedly, a degree of cirrhosis of the liver.

'This looks bad. It will need a Hartmann's procedure. Should not take too long though,' David told his anaesthetist.

'OK but he does not have much of a blood pressure so pronto please, Mr. Sellu.'

A Hartmann's procedure is when the lowest part of the colon above the rectum, the sigmoid colon, is removed. A colostomy is made upstream and the top of the rectum below is sewn over. By this means, there is no danger of a leak from a join-up, an anastomosis, as there is not one. The faeces are collected in a bag until one day, when the patient is fit again, the colon and rectum can be reconstructed with another major operation.

Sellu continued resecting the sigmoid colon but encountered quite a lot of bleeding. Finally the operation was over and a colostomy fashioned. At 1am Mr. Hughes was transferred to the Intensive Care Unit and David finally managed to get home.

During the next three days Mr. Hughes fought for his life with the constant attention of the ICU team.

But he did not make it.

He died at about 4pm on Sunday the 14th February.

***

I heard about David Sellu's case the next week and reflected on the fact that, as a colorectal surgeon, I had lost plenty of patients with sepsis from perforations. It was well known that up to one third of patients with this type of peritonitis do not survive. I also knew that the speed of getting the patient to theatre does not alter the prognosis all that much.

What happened in the following few months surprised us all. An investigation launched by the Clementine Churchill Hospital by a pathologist and a surgeon not only looked into the case of Mr. Hughes but investigated several previous cases that David Sellu had operated upon. From thousands of patients he had treated at this private hospital, they found two cases that they noted might have been managed differently. But none of these had been flagged up as worrying at the time.

Their report was critical of David Sellu's handling of the case. Following this report David Sellu was suspended from the Clementine Churchill Hospital in September 2010, but a General Medical Council hearing later in October of the same year concluded that there was 'no case to answer' concerning Sellu's treatment of Mr. Hughes.

In October 2010, the coroner's inquest into Mr. Hughes' death took place. David found to his surprise that he was being sharply cross-examined by the coroner and was unprepared for this criticism. Questions about whether he had prescribed antibiotics and, whether he had looked at the CT scans, were asked. To David's surprise he was commanded to leave the court. Forty minutes later, he was informed by one of his sons, who had accompanied him to the court that the coroner was to refer the case to the police, as he suspected a crime had been committed.

Sometime during this process the Crown Prosecution Service took the unprecedented step of appointing a second expert witness. The first, a respected professor of surgery, had concluded there was no negligence in Sellu's handling of Mr. Hughes. The second, a retired surgeon, Michael Kelly, whose reputation was not that of the professor, saw it differently.

This led to a further GMC investigation following which restrictive conditions were placed on David Sellu's work at Ealing Hospital, his NHS base. He was informed that he must expect to be questioned by the police. What followed were several bruising interviews and, finally, a charge of manslaughter being levelled at David Sellu in July 2012.

When I heard that the case had become a criminal investigation, I was puzzled. If David Sellu was to be placed in the dock, then every general surgeon in the land should be in there with him. Death was an expected complication of the disease processes that present to surgeons as emergencies. If we are lucky, we can save some but not all.

Of course, hindsight is a wonderful thing. We can look back at any case and say it might have been better if we had done this, or that, or nothing at all. It goes without saying that, if David Sellu had been able to operate earlier that day, he would have done so. Though it was more than likely it would not have changed the outcome at all.

When I was in training, a wise old surgeon once remarked that we all had skeletons in our cupboards. Patients we would like to have treated differently. The story of William dying of his perforated gall bladder in Chapter 13 is a perfect illustration of one of mine.

But here was a case of Sellu doing the right thing, with what appeared to be unavoidable delay, and the police were involved?

When David was suspended from the private hospital I took over his post as surgical representative on the Medical Advisory Board of the Clementine Churchill Hospital. In addition, because I saw the danger of working under an unsupportive management team in the hospital, I also took myself off the emergency surgery rota that I had set up for the hospital fifteen years before. I wanted to protect myself but also by being on the board I wanted to understand what had happened to him.

The process was slow and inexorable with catastrophic consequences for the surgeon who had tried to operate to save Mr. Hughes' life.

Unbelievably, David Sellu was convicted at the Old Bailey of gross negligence manslaughter of his patient Mr. Hughes in November 2013. He was sentenced to two and a half years in prison. David Sellu's conviction sent shock waves through the medical profession. Surgeons, particularly, began talking of finding a safer profession to pursue. Some even decided to throw in the towel. I met one young, brilliant female consultant colorectal surgeon who left the profession directly because of the Sellu case.

I wrote to David in prison, initially Belmarsh, the high security prison, to try to understand more but his polite but depressed replies did not enlighten me. As time wore on I discovered there were several of us unable to square the circle of this sad affair. The Friends of David Sellu group was formed by Ian Franklin, a vascular surgeon, and we started to raise money for an appeal. We also wished to raise the profession's understanding of what, we were quite sure, was a gross miscarriage of justice.

Dr. Jenny Vaughan, a consultant neurologist, who like me was puzzled by Sellu's predicament, spearheaded the medico-legal defence. Her forensic brain and her tireless search for the truth focused our campaign. She looked again at all the circumstances of the investigation and the trial. She galvanized a new team of lawyers to assist David.

The Friends of David Sellu began to get up a head of steam. We arranged fund-raising dinners and the money flowed in. Ian Franklin and I organised public meetings. I wrote articles in the medical press while Jenny Vaughan mobilised many of David Sellu's grateful patients and admiring colleagues through social media. She also conducted a survey of doctors nationwide as to how the case, and others like it, may have adversely affected the way they practise medicine. Her findings made disturbing reading.

Sadly, our professional bodies were supine in defence of David Sellu. Although the medical defence organisation that David belonged to, the Medical Protection Society, was supportive, they had failed him, to some extent, as they had omitted to appoint a criminal barrister to defend him. Rather they relied on a medical negligence barrister to represent him at his trial. It seems that this barrister had been significantly wrong-footed at Sellu's criminal trial.

The British Medical Association, the Royal Colleges of Surgeons and the Association of Coloproctology were all found wanting in their support. Sellu was a member of all of these organisations but they offered no real help or counselling.

As the months wore on the new legal team, spurred on by Jenny Vaughan, mounted a leave to appeal which succeeded on its second attempt. Finally a full Appeal Court hearing was agreed to.

It was suggested that I might be an expert witness for the Sellu case but, as I knew Sellu prior to 2010, I would be seen as having a conflict of interest. In consequence, of that decision I managed to persuade one of my younger colleagues at St. Mark's, Professor Omar Faiz, to be the expert for this new legal challenge. He was nervous at first, as this was a new field of endeavour for him, but he excelled in his task. His analysis of the nature of the Hughes' case was a major factor in the final outcome.

Meanwhile, Sellu had served half his sentence of two-and-a-half years and was out of prison on licence. He talked at dinners and at open meetings. He was a focus of much interest within the profession. His quiet humility, his stoicism and his measured approach to the disaster that had befallen him was widely admired.

Perhaps, a more aggressive approach in defending himself against the accusation of manslaughter might have been more effective in countering the police investigation. Pointing out just how complex decision-making in medicine is, and not being so trusting in the ability of the criminal justice system to come to a fair and rational conclusion, might have served him better. We know the criminal court was swayed by the dogmatic tone from the expert for the prosecution, Michael Kelly. He succeeded in persuading the jury that David Sellu was an outlier among surgeons in the way had managed the case. This was plainly rubbish in the opinion of almost all practising surgeons.

A less gentlemanly response from Sellu's defence team might have been more effective in an English criminal court where the adversarial ethos is so much part of the mix. Sellu's trusting and passive response to the charges against him is one of the reasons that I now believe that racism unconsciously played a part in his conviction. Until his case, I had always believed in the impartiality of the English legal system and the General Medical Council, the body that polices the medical profession.

On paper, these organisations are set up to be impartial, but I now think that they are subliminally racist. They do not take into account that some individuals cannot defend themselves against charges as well as others. How else can we explain the extraordinarily high proportion of BAME doctors and nurses in the struck-off, sanctioned or criminally charged group in our society?

Jenny Vaughan and the new legal team, supported anew by the Medical Protection Society, were now ready for the Appeal Court. I was only able to get away from my work at Northwick Park Hospital for one of the days of Sellu's Appeal at the Royal Courts of Justice in Fleet Street. I remember that day sitting below the three distinguished judges, chaired by Sir Brian Leveson, when the chairman said to the two barristers in front of him:

'Of course, learned colleagues, it must be acknowledged that the test of criminal negligence or manslaughter ought to be different for doctors, and particularly surgeons, than for the general population as half of the surgeons' patients are dying already. This certainly was true in this case.'

It was after I heard that statement that I knew David Sellu would be exonerated in the Appeal Court judgement.

And so he was.

On the 15th of November 2016, just a little under seven years from those fateful few days in 2010, the Appeal Court judges declared:

'We have come to the clear conclusion that the way in which the issue of gross negligence was approached (and, in particular, the consequential direction to the jury) was inadequate. As a result, the conviction is unsafe and is quashed.'

A miscarriage of justice had been righted. Sellu had suffered imprisonment for a clinical scenario that all general surgeons experience regularly.

But this was not the end of it for David Sellu. The Medical Practitioners Tribunal Service (MPTS) insisted it go through all the evidence again. I once wrote cheekily that the MPTS is the military wing of the GMC. So it seemed as it sifted through the case, line by line, again. The MPTS had found yet another surgical expert willing who, with the benefit of hindsight, was willing to say how he might have treated Mr. Hughes better. David Sellu, with Jenny Vaughan and Omar Faiz behind him, would have to battle it all out again.

But, this time the balance of power had changed and the Sellu team were briefed and ready. It took no more than a day to restore David to the Medical Register.

David Sellu's actions in February 2010 were finally vindicated. But his career had been destroyed.

***

In 2015, David Sellu came to work alongside me at St. Mark's Hospital as an honorary consultant surgeon. My hospital was willing to give him a second chance while his appeals were being heard. That was a credit to our temporary medical director Dr. Charles Cayley as other institutions were keen to avoid any risk.

Sellu's desire to get back into theatre had faded, so he came once a week to see some of my outpatients in a room next to mine. We would share the cases and discuss what we would advise the patients. As I expected he was meticulous, courteous and kindly and the patients loved seeing him. When I had first got to know him properly, for the first time, after his release from prison, he had been very depressed but now he was beginning to smile again.

Although his experiences in prison were degrading, he had come out with his dignity intact but with not much to laugh about. Over the four years that we have worked quietly together, I have heard him laugh more and more and seen his broad smile brighten up our consulting rooms.

Part of the process of recovery for David was to write about his tribulations. In his book *Did He Save Lives?* can be found a detailed and moving account of his life inside and outside prison. It deserves to be read by many. It is not a book full of bitterness though there is much sadness within its pages. It is also an important story of a death of a patient, whose family's mourning cannot have been helped by the inappropriate prosecution that followed.

Did He Save Lives? is about how a doctor was wronged but won through in the end. It explains how complex the issues in medical cases are and how our actions as doctors can be so easily misunderstood and criticised after the event. David has taken this message to the British medical profession and others by lecturing all over the country. He has spoken to packed lecture halls.

With his book I hope he will also have spread this message all over the world as many doctors overseas wondered, in horror, how the English justice system had engineered such a misadventure.

I did not know David Sellu much at all until February 2010. He was just a fellow consultant at a hospital where I worked who I had met in the corridor once or twice. I remember feeling a touch of envy when I heard the nurses on the wards saying how that nice David Sellu had been there and how many presents his patients had given him that week. I did not know then that he would play a substantial role in my life in the years that followed that winter night in February 2010.

As a writer I have often found important causes to scribble about. I have sometimes been proud of my small contributions to the debates. However, the efforts I made, as one of the Friends of David Sellu, has given me more fulfilment than almost anything else I have put my pen to. I was willing to join battle against one of my indirect employers, the Clementine Churchill Hospital. By doing so I risked part of my livelihood as I publicly criticised the organisation that I considered had targetted a consultant to cover their own shortcomings. I stuck my neck out when I realised a miscarriage of justice had taken place. I am glad that I did.

The Clementine Churchill Hospital has almost certainly suffered from the bad publicity of the Sellu case. The disgust in the profession, as to how he was treated, was widespread. I know of several consultants who did not apply for admitting rights at the hospital, and steered their patients to other more supportive competitors. In that sense, the hospital got what it deserved. They tried to scapegoat one of their consultants instead of trying to understand the condition that led to Mr. Hughes' death or admitting the hospital's own deficiencies, such as the lack of a rota of emergency anaesthetists.

They might have taken sanctions against me as I stood against them in public meetings, TV interviews and in articles. They were wise to avoid a fight. I would have welcomed this as I would have fought back aggressively and given them as good as they gave me. But that was not the case. Instead they kept silent.

In my files is a copy of a letter I wrote to the Clementine Churchill Hospital in 2008, two years before the Sellu case. In the letter I called for the setting up of an anaesthetic rota on safety grounds. I will keep that document safe.

At the beginning of this chapter I noted that doctors, and particularly surgeons, are subject today to much criticism. It is thought that up to a third of doctors will be reported to the GMC during their medical lifetime. All will suffer greatly from this unpleasant process but only a tiny minority will be sanctioned. I have not been spared the GMC's attention. Two decades ago, I was reported, along with seven other colleagues, by a disgruntled anaesthetist, who none of us wanted to work with. The criticisms were fanciful and spurious. The complaint was seen as vexatious and thrown out very promptly. However it was a sobering exercise and one I would not like to repeat. Not surprisingly the GMC's reputation within the profession is at an all-time low.

***

Sellu's story is of one of a distinguished, caring surgeon who came to our shores because of his special talents, but who was mistreated by the system, and whose last fifteen years of practice was lost to our country. In David Sellu's case, unjustified criticism led to the destruction of his career. In consequence, fewer will choose to stay in the profession.

If the excessive censure of the medical profession multiplies further, I judge that right-minded, intelligent young men and women will find other less risky ways to occupy their lives.

They will certainly be reluctant to follow their predecessors.

This will be to the detriment of all of us who one day will be patients ourselves.

Chapter 22: Covid-19

❖

I was skiing with Christina and a few close friends in the Italian Dolomites in late January 2020 when I first heard about a new disease spreading across the world from the city of Wuhan in China. The snow was clean and fresh and the hotel in the smart mountain town of Madonna di Campiglio was perfect. The mountain food was delizioso with the dense vino rosso of the Veneto wine region slipping down merrily after a long day on the pistes. Thoughts of a new world plague could not have been further from our minds.

It was said that an epidemic was rapidly advancing westward. It was a dangerous form of a well-known minor enemy that was recognised to be one of the many causes of the common cold, the coronavirus. The name struck a chord in my mind as I remembered this regal sounding virus from my medical school days. So this was another new nasty form of a well-known relatively innocuous organism? I remembered that SARS and MERS a couple of decades before had also been coronaviruses but they had petered out quite quickly.

Just that week the new virus had been rechristened 'Covid-19' by the World Health Organisation, as if by giving it a new name we were acknowledging its newfound virulence. Whether it had emerged from a bat sold at a wet market in Wuhan, or from a research laboratory nearby, was not yet known.

When I returned home a few days later, I pulled from the bookshelf the microbiology textbook that I had bought in my first year as a medical student at University College London. Published in 1969, its dry, old pages contained on page 174 a paragraph about those organisms known to produce coryza, the common cold.

Organ culture of material from colds led to the discovery of small RNA viruses which have envelopes resembling myxoviruses - named coronaviruses. Production of vaccines that will prevent colds seems a long way off.

As my ultra-violet suntan from the high mountains began to fade, the World Health Organisation declared that Covid-19 was now the causative organism of this global pandemic. Suddenly there was talk of quarantine and the unfamiliar terms of 'social distancing' and 'self-isolation' were splashed over the front pages of newspapers and internet search engines.

By mid-March not much yet had changed in England. The Festival of National Hunt Racing at Cheltenham took place on March 10th. Some said it should have been cancelled. Perhaps they were right for it later emerged that several cases of Covid-19 were contracted at that meeting. There was now talk of banning all public gatherings. For Christina and I, our final act of freedom was a week before Prime Minister Boris Johnson locked down the whole country on Monday 16th March. We attended a concert at the Royal Albert Hall given by the London Musical Theatre Orchestra under the baton of Freddie Tapner. It was a magical evening of song delivered by top West End stars.

I remember noticing quite a few people in front of us were coughing loudly throughout the performance. I later learnt that several aerosol particles of Covid-19 were shared that night and many fell ill. That evening Christina and I were just bumping elbows with our acquaintances in the new normal style. Fortunately we were well out of range of the rising droplets shimmering above the audience below us as the spotlights illuminated the quite brilliant vocal stars.

I hope no-one died who went to the Albert Hall that night.

The fear was now real and universal. This previously benign fragment of RNA was spreading rapidly and country after country locked down their populations. Britain was a week or two behind others, taking the pragmatic approach to a crisis, while trying to keep the country in business for as long as possible. However, this laissez faire approach may have cost more lives in the long run as the death rate in the UK rose rapidly to become the highest in Europe.

Suddenly everything changed. We were transported to the 1950s. The skies above rural Hertfordshire were gloriously empty of jet airliners and the International Space Station twinkled brightly as we followed it racing across the sky each evening. The country lanes were filled with cyclists in lycra exercising vigorously and there were strange city-shaped walkers everywhere. Presumably they were all out from London enjoying the peace of the more rural shires. Locked down with three of our four children and a miscellaneous boyfriend our lockdown routines became most enjoyable. It was a long way from the misery unfolding elsewhere.

I had more time to ride Galway my chestnut gelding. When the world seemed half-mad with fear I would go into the fields and hug him. It is said that the outside of a horse is good for the inside of a man. So it was with me and my Irish equine friend at that uncertain time.

At my place of work it was a different story.

***

Northwick Park Hospital was nearly overwhelmed with breathless patients. Within three weeks six hundred beds were filled with Covid-19 cases. All cases except emergency medicine, obstetric deliveries and surgery were cancelled. Cancer patients were treated in a private hospital in Central London. Benign urgent cases were transferred to the Clementine Churchill Hospital nearby that had agreed to support the NHS effort and was deemed a 'clean' Covid-19-free site. Nightingale Hospitals prefabricated specially for Covid-19 patients were being set up all over the country to cope with the expected demand.

Back at Northwick Park seventy ventilators were pumping away day and night as the killer cold took hold of the obese, black and ethnic minorities, the co-morbid and the elderly. The only stroke of luck for the planet was the odd fact that this pandemic was killing mostly those who had benefitted from many years of life. In this way it was completely different from the bubonic plague of the fourteenth and sixteenth centuries, which had killed 30-50% of the population, wiping out all ages indiscriminately. The Spanish influenza pandemic of 1918 was even more malign, as it had specifically targetted the young, leaving twenty million dead.

Generously my younger colleagues had taken me off the emergency rota as I was now in my late sixties. Despite feeling I was not contributing as much as I should be, I did not argue. I filled much of my time conducting telephone clinics and triaging those that needed to be seen face-to-face urgently. It would be four months before I was operating routinely again.

I learnt the ritual of attending what became known as the 'donning room' where I was fitted and trained for the different types of PPE (personal protective equipment). I learnt what Scott Safety and JSP Jetstream hoods were. I struggled slipping FFP3 on and then testing it with a 'fit test'. These were all new and unpleasant rituals and when we dispensed with the equipment at the end of a procedure we would do something called 'doffing'. Evidently the coronavirus was important enough to have its own language.

As the warm summer of 2020 wore on the burden of wearing this equipment became intolerable with medical and nursing staff having to take regular breaks to cool down and wipe off the sweat. Several brave younger colleagues, many surgeons and physicians, volunteered to help in the Intensive Care Department under the supervision of intensivists and infectious diseases consultants. It was a case of everyone pulling together. There was a war time feel to it all as the country clapped every Thursday evening for their NHS heroes.

During that time these heroes were often witness to terrible tragedies as many of their patients died very quickly.

An average of five days from start of the symptoms to admission.

Five more days to complete breathlessness and death on a ventilator.

This misery was compounded as relatives of the dying were largely excluded from contact with their loved ones for fear of further spread of the virus.

Even bodies in morgues were not allowed visitors.

Not that they would notice.

Many of my medical and nursing friends got infected. They bravely battled against this deadly slice of RNA. Extreme fatigue, muscle pains, loss of taste, persisting cough, high fever and breathlessness were the main symptoms. Most sweated it out at home with the help of spouses while others were completely isolated and horribly alone in their flats and apartments. The most breathless were forced to go to hospital hoping, but dreading, to be admitted. If they were taken into the Covid-19 wards they were placed alongside other patients fighting for their lives or simply sent back home being told they were not yet ill enough to merit admission.

The doctors soon got familiar with the tell-tale chest signs of Covid-19 infection on their CT scans. They copied their Chinese colleagues by putting memorable names to the appearances of those images. Pure ground glass opacity, parallel pleura sign, paving stone sign, halo sign and the reversed halo sign. Never in the history of medicine had so much medical effort been applied so rapidly to one disease. Even by the 20th March 2020, one hundred and sixty-five papers had been published on the subject. By the 10th August 2020, 13,453,361 tests for Covid-19 had been conducted in the UK alone. By early November 2020, there had been 34 million cases of Covid-19 documented worldwide with more than a million deaths. A mortality rate of 3%. By the end of January 2021 there had been over 100,000 deaths in the UK and two million deaths world-wide. But by the spring a successful vaccination programme and a second lockdown had successfully brought the infection under control in the UK. However by April the epicentre of the pandemic had migrated again with Brazil and India in dire straits. A new delta variant had emerged and was ready to continue the chaos.

Amidst all this activity there were piteous tragedies near to home involving those I had worked with. The oldest consultant surgeon still working at Northwick Park, Raj Bhutiani, who had operated alongside me since I arrived at the hospital, got ill early in April. He was quickly admitted and ventilated. His dreadful journey through the NHS first took him to Harefield Heart Hospital and then to the

Brompton Chest Hospital in central London. I sent messages of support to his family who assured us that he was fighting hard but still needing ventilation for long periods through a tracheostomy. Raj was a fighter but the virus won in the end and he died after an eleven-month struggle in mid-February 2021.

His personal tragedy was being echoed throughout the world. If the virus did not kill you it wreaked vengeance in more subtle ways. We heard that the first post-Covid-19 lung transplant had been carried out on a 29-year old in the United States. The chronic effects of Covid-19 on the lungs, heart, brain and kidneys was more and more being recognized, so-called 'Long Covid'.

Mirroring my poor colleague's plight was the case of Dr. Alfa Saadu. Retired from the NHS, he took up the call to come and help with the Covid-19 emergency. Quickly he fell sick and died. I had been a fellow student with Alfa at University College London fifty years before. I remember him as a clever Nigerian who was able to contribute as a doctor both in his native Sub-Saharan Africa and in the UK.

But if these good doctors' deaths were unfair, the fate of Dr. Erwin Spannagl was even more shocking. Erwin was German and was a fit fifty-eight year old. He had worked with us at Northwick Park for the last twenty years. For ten years he covered the hospital as a registrar in general surgery. Often he and I would be sharing difficult cases together at night or weekends. More recently the vascular team had needed his surgical skills so he had worked as an associate specialist supporting them. He was pleasant, committed to his patients and exceptionally hard working.

Going through a difficult divorce had made Erwin a little depressed in recent years but, when I last bumped into him in the corridor in early February 2020, I noticed he was a lot more cheerful. I knew he lived in a suburb of Potsdam near the German capital and occasionally I would quiz him about it. I learnt of its importance to German history being the seat of Prussian kings and, until 1918, of the last German Kaizer. We often talked of the meticulous renovation he was conducting on his nineteenth century house there. His routine had been to fly over to London and live in the on-call rooms when he was on duty and then fly home again. He never had a base in Harrow, always relying on hospital accommodation at Northwick Park.

He first developed symptoms of Covid-19 while working on the ICU at the hospital. His job in the unit had been to provide vascular access in the form of arterial and venous lines for the sickest patients. It was in this overcrowded inner sanctum at Northwick Park that he caught the coronavirus from a patient. This is pertinent when I consider what happened in the next few days.

Recognising he was ill, he informed the hospital. They ordered him to cease work and self-isolate, adding that he should vacate the on-call rooms and rent somewhere locally. How easy would that have been when you are ill and far from home and your loved ones? Ignoring this harsh advice he flew home on the 25th of March 2020 from Stansted Airport to Berlin and corralled himself in his house in Potsdam. Preventing his two daughters from visiting to avoid getting infected he sweated it out alone.

His body was found two days later.

The shock to the surgical team was immense but the hospital took three months to acknowledge the fact. It seemed that those in high places were more interested in the fact that he had ignored the risks to others and flown home. No proper obituary notice or condolence note was published by the hospital until early October 2020 nearly six months later. It was left to one of our vascular consultants Tahir Hussein to raise a condolence fund and send it, with a sad note, to his poor grieving daughters.

This painful story was compounded in our national press by The Guardian newspaper publishing an account quoting the Mayor of Potsdam's outrage.

'As a doctor he knew the risk of infection. How could he then go on to mingle among the crowds in several countries? The man was acting completely irresponsibly.'

But I wonder what would you have done?
You are alone.

You are ill in a foreign country wondering whether you might have the virus. It had not been confirmed by any test and was, at that time, of uncertain virulence and infectivity. By this time in late March 2020, the pandemic had not yet been fully characterized, and its real dangers not entirely appreciated.

You have been refused accommodation by the hospital that has directly employed and then indirectly infected you.

I would argue that most of us would have high-tailed back to our home to be near our loved ones and self-isolate there.

And that is what poor Erwin did.

And it was there that he died with his friends and family hearing nothing but criticism rather than sympathy for a brave doctor lost in his prime, working hard to help his patients.

To illustrate how I was thinking at that time I will take the liberty to quote from the scribblings of Mr. Slop, my nom de plume, outlining his life in his imaginary hospital beset by Covid–19, somewhere in Middle England:

It was certainly true that Midshire Hospital Trust with its three hospitals in the county had been a hell-hole for a few weeks. Mr. Slop FRCS had lost two colleagues and a third was suffering his fifth-week unconscious on a ventilator. Slop had never been in the armed forces so had never lost friends in action before. When he got home to his rural retreat, his mood was more sombre than his wife could ever remember.

However, there had been some respite from the misery. One of Slop's junior colleagues had serenaded a recovering patient out of the ICU with his expert violin playing and had made national TV. The hospital was giving free coffee and car parking to its staff and there was a feeling of 'we are all in this together' that Slop, who was a post-war baby boomer, had never quite felt before. Even the humour being propagated through the internet was of superior quality and the 25% discount off take-aways for NHS staff was worth a few bob.

(Courtesy of The Bulletin of The Royal College of Surgeons of England)

***

Week by week the lockdown continued and economies around the world ground to a halt.

Some people got depressed.

Others frustrated.

Some ate too much.

Others exercised in the dark as night-walkers.

Conspiracy theories were all around. Ignorance and fear were common currency.

By July 2020, the hospitals I worked in slowly began to empty of Covid-19 patients as the incidence of the infection began to fall. But the beds were still largely empty as few non-Covid patients were being treated. The corridors were deserted and the carparks half-full.

There seemed to be no winners in all this.

***

That was until I met Corinne James and her husband.

It was Friday afternoon and I was conducting a mini-clinic in the private hospital. It was a mixture of private and NHS 'Choose and Book' patients. Mostly it was a virtual clinic conducted on the telephone but at 2.30pm I saw Mrs. James face-to-face, or rather mask-to-mask.

'I have come to see you in desperation Mr. McDonald as my neighbour said you were the best person in the hospital and you would be able to help me!'

'Maybe you need to get neighbours with better judgement,' I joked, trying to diffuse the obvious tension.

I could see how fraught she was.

'Joking aside just tell me what the problem is.'

'Well, I was quite all right until three weeks ago and then I got constipated and bloated. I have this pain in my lower belly and my back. I just don't feel well anymore and usually I am very active.'

I glanced up at her over my reading glasses and saw a woman in distress. Although she did not seem undernourished she looked pasty and had a very worried look on her face.

'The GPs said they could not see me at this time of Covid-19 so we went to Accident & Emergency where this young doctor said it was a urinary tract infection and prescribed antibiotics.'

'Did anyone examine you properly?' I asked.

'Not at all,' she replied. 'Sometimes I wonder if I am imagining it all. But I weighed myself yesterday and find I have lost five kilograms in just three weeks.'

I then took a history from her and learnt that she had been completely fit until three weeks prior to the symptoms coming on and then all this had happened. That made my ears prick up. I often ask my medical students if cancer has a long history or a short one. They usually say long history. They are wrong. It has a relatively short history. If a patient tells me they have had a symptom for two years they have not got cancer unless it is a co-incidental event. If they tell me that their abdominal pain or their difficulty in swallowing has only been with them six weeks I am much more worried.

Although three weeks is a very short period for cancer symptoms to present to the doctor it was a definite possibility. Inflammation presents in the first one to five days. Cancer occupies the middle ground between a few weeks and a few months only. It is the same for almost any part of the body. The lump in the neck that has been there for three years will be a benign multi-nodular goitre. But a lump only noticed four weeks ago, as it was in Christina's case in Chapter 4, is a different matter.

I examined Corinne in the presence of her husband. Her abdomen was a bit doughy but there were no masses palpable. It was quite distended and dull when I tapped it suggesting fluid or solid elements rather than lots of wind or flatus.

'Now I must examine you down below,' I said. 'It's the way a bowel surgeon like me says hello,' I joked again.

Corinne smiled weakly.

'OK I understand,' she added.

I then performed a rectal examination. The lower rectum and anus felt fine but in front I could feel a mass between my index finger and the vagina. Was that hard stool or something else? I judged the latter. When the examination was over and the patient was back in her seat with her mask on I gave her my opinion.

'I think something is going on here and I am going to get a scan straight away and a few blood tests.'

Because of Covid-19 and its effect on the hospital I knew the CT scanner would be available without the necessity of any wait. A quick telephone call to the radiographer and the scan was arranged along with the blood test. Less than an hour later I was sitting in the darkened radiologists' room with Dr. Miranda Harvie looking at Corinne's scans. I was pleased it was Miranda as I had a high regard for her opinion. This New Zealander was always such an enthusiastic, helpful and caring radiologist. She would get to the bottom of Corinne's problem I was sure.

The miracle of imaging in today's world is truly beyond description. When I was a medical student we could palpate and percuss (tap) chests and abdomens. We could listen to the bowel sounds and then we could just guess what was wrong. Today we can slice through the patient, centimetre by centimetre, without hurting them. Then flick another switch and the computers can reconstruct the images into two dimensions and now into three dimensions. Some can go so far as to do 3D printing.

Almost nothing can hide and radiologists like Miranda, who organise and interpret these scans, truly have eyes in the back of their heads. They miss nothing.

'Well, Peter, I am afraid it's not good news. Ascites, fluid in the abdomen, and omental secondaries arising probably from the left ovary.'

What Miranda was telling me, was that Corinne had Stage III ovarian cancer. Bad though it was at least I now had a diagnosis to work on. Although it was outside my area of expertise, I had seen plenty before. I knew I had to find a gynaecologist to see her soon.

Without giving me a moment longer to think the situation through, Miranda continued:

'I know just the right gynaecology oncologist at Queen Charlotte's to get her to see.'

Within an hour I had phoned Professor Christina Fotopoulou who like Miranda was both helpful and charming. Next morning Corinne was in her consulting rooms and I got a text back from the good professor.

Dear Mr. McDonald

Hope you are well. I saw Corinne the day after we talked and as you had noted she was indeed very symptomatic. I arranged her immediate admission and we drained 8 litres of ascites. Her albumin was very low at 14 and the CRP had increased to 300 with a leucocytosis also, so all that in combination with her very extensive disease made primary surgery with extensive stripping very risky, especially with all the issues of the pandemic and the limited ITU beds etc..

That is why we started her on some chemotherapy, after a biopsy that confirmed high grade serous ovarian cancer, to make her disease a bit more amenable to surgery. As she was dry we rehydrated her and gave her some protein nutrition and antibiotics and I will operate on her after 3 cycles. I will update you again after the surgery.

She is doing so far much better, feels stronger and her CRP and white cell counts have gone down and her albumin is increasing.

I just also wanted to let you know that she was extremely grateful to you for your advice and care and that you managed to organise everything so quickly for her.

Also from my side thank you so much for referring her to me.
Hope you have a good summer.
Very best wishes

Professor Fotopoulou

PS despite the peritoneal dissemination if we get her macroscopically tumour free and consolidate with more chemo her five-year survival is around 65%. Not great but still better than some other cancers.

It is for moments like these that I work, and that I will miss, when I will inevitably have to retire. Although I had personally done very little for Corinne, she saw it differently.

I had listened to her story and not just fobbed her off.

I could hear this was a new and real problem that had arisen. Not a urinary tract infection.

Something much more sinister which needed a quick diagnosis and a firm hand to get it under control.

With Miranda's help, I had found that firm hand.

If anyone could get Corinne's tumour under control, it would be that Greek professor.

***

A physician once said to me that he had chosen to be a physician and not a surgeon because he could not countenance changing into theatre scrubs and wearing a mask every day.

But now in 2021, everyone wears a mask. Quite often they wear scrubs and gowns too. Even between second and third waves of Covid-19, when we are allowed to go to restaurants, we can hear only a muffled menu and a whispered wine list.

A futuristic nightmare.

It is all an unpleasant dream.

***

But dreams never last.

Time inevitably puts a stop to them.

As I put on my jacket after a face-to-face masked clinic and head for my car for the drive back to Hertfordshire, I curse Covid-19 and the nightmares it has initiated.

The empty wards.

The dead doctors and nurses.

The full crematoria.
The postponed weddings.
The failing economy.
The burgeoning domestic violence.
The holidays postponed.
All that is true.

But as I look up at the sky above my house each evening all is clear. I can see Venus already visible even though the semi-darkness. The air is clean, the roads free of traffic and the world around me noiseless. The moon is full and more sharply defined than I have ever seen it.

This is, in part at least, a better dream and not just a nightmare.

And so was that quick CT scan that afforded a speedy diagnosis, referral and early treatment of Corinne James that may yet save her life. Spared the virus, she was now embarking on a hard and painful journey. With Covid-19's empty scanner and with Miranda's help I had been able to treat her better than in more usual times.

At least, just this once, the new-normal had served me well.

Chapter 23:
Retirement And Beyond

❖

Humans as they age look back at their earliest years with rose-tinted glasses. So much was better then. So much has changed for the worse. It was not like that in my day.

The benefit of a long career means I can truthfully look back and make a judgement.

I began this memoir with patient H365271 dying in the early 1990s of stab wounds on my operating table. It was a drug-related, gang-inspired homicide. The man was attacked close to one of the hospitals I work in.

Meaningless.

Tragic.

Stupid.

That death on the table was at the very beginning of the thirty years I have worked at Northwick Park Hospital.

This very week, as I write this final chapter, a 17-year boy was stabbed to death in broad daylight on the footpath leading to the tube station at Northwick Park Hospital. My secretary, who had been with me on the day of that first murder, had walked that same path home just ten minutes prior to the youth being found. I know no details of this second senseless killing but I expect it too was a drug-related, gang-inspired homicide.

Meaningless.

Tragic.

Stupid.

Life goes on much as it has before.

Some things get better.

Some things get worse.

Much stays the same.

***

After being born and getting married it could be said that retiring from full-time employment is the third most important milestone of an individual life. Death is the fourth and is usually non-negotiable.

Out of these four moments of destiny only two are under our direct control. It is clear that in regard to the decision to marry many make the wrong choice. Unhappiness and divorce may follow. I certainly made this wrong choice but was rescued by marrying Christina, a person I could get along with, build a family together and love deeply.

But do we also make wrong decisions about when to retire? Throughout the years of work, retirement is talked about as a goal to be anticipated with great eagerness. We contribute to our pensions and we are given projected earnings in retirement but many do not think about the consequences of leaving work behind.

Why do we want to retire?

Presumably to be relieved of the stresses of getting up early, shaved and ready for the day? To be free of the difficult decision-making or the tedium that our employment brings? To put one's feet up and spend more time watching the wind rustle through the autumn leaves? To enjoy doing those things that we have always wanted to do?

But this assumes that work is bad and retirement always good. What if work is stimulating and retirement boring? What if giving up work is relinquishing something that we have spent years fighting for? Retirement is often a sudden loss of status. I worked fiercely hard to become a doctor and then a surgeon.

When I retire that is all gone in a moment.

The decision is also completely irreversible in most instances.

And what about pay? Some wit said that retirement is half the pay and twice the wife.

And what about that all too important relationship with the spouse? Another wag said that they married their partner for life but not for lunch. I read recently that divorce's second peak is around retirement. In America the divorce rate for people aged 50 and above has doubled since the 1990s. For people aged 65 and above, it has tripled.

There are some serious points behind these slick quips and statistics. I have spent much of my life earning money to balance the budget to look after myself, my wife and my children. Suddenly I take the biggest pay cut of the century by retiring. Being a bit of an investor I have always looked at ways to make my savings grow. Property? Shares? Savings Accounts? Extra pension contributions? Mostly they provide disappointing returns. Quite often I have lost money.

Then suddenly I take the worse financial decision of my life and retire? Half the pay? Maybe less? If I lost half my equity in a property deal I would think it a very bad investment indeed. But when I retire I do not lose it just once. I forfeit 50% again year-after-year-after-year.

There is the assumption that retirement must be better than working. That the disciplines, that work has taught us, will follow us into retirement. But will they? Sloppy habits are easy to acquire when no-one is looking. I may be tempted to miss a shave and to start the alcohol clock at lunchtime rather than of an evening. When the sun is over the yard arm rather than at four bells, as my ex-Royal Marine father might have said.

And what about all those wonderful holidays I will be able to take when I retire? That does not always work out either. In lockdown this year many retirees must feel cheated, as they have been cooped up like fugitives hiding from an invading army.

Actually I have enough holidays already. I do not need to travel more. I did all that in spades when I was young. And if I did holiday more, the cost of holidays in retirement might suddenly become a factor. I know plenty of retired friends who have run out of money living the high life.

Until very recently the world concluded that the default factor was to retire while you still had capacity. But what about the idea of keeping the brain working and the body moving to retain capacity?

And that nagging thought of being able to avoid dementia? The challenges of work certainly might do that. Suduko and bridge can be a substitute, but I have seen men and women quickly fade to nothing when they pull on their slippers and give up the day job.

And what if I enjoy most of aspects of my work and I am still fit enough to do them? Of course, there are some repetitive moments.

Waiting around in theatre for the cases to start.

Consulting with a patient who wants to burden me with every detail of an imaginary ailment.

Performing some meaningless, management-demanded task to complete my accreditation.

True, these are all frustrating moments.

But on the other hand, if I retire I lose those instances of great elation.

The pleasure of teaching the students and seeing how excited they are learning the skills that will take them forward in their careers.

Assisting a young surgeon through a complex operation? A pleasure almost without parallel.

Seeing the smile on the patient's face when they go home happy and cured.

Receiving notification that the bank has received my salary each month and that I can pay for the next indulgence without worry.

These pleasures will all be lost when I retire. I will become an ex-surgeon, an emeritus doctor, an aging retiree waiting for the inevitable. At least, while still at work, I can delude myself that the grim reaper might take others first as I am still useful.

A retired ex-colleague said to me not so long ago:

'Of course, Peter you are too scared to retire. You should try it. It's really good. I have never looked back.'

Well, he cannot look back. He cannot go back even if he wished. Not to the high profile job he had as clinical director and professor. But when I asked his wife what she thought, she mumbled something about not being able to go to the supermarket without the professor supervising her.

My identical twin brother, an architect, retired eight years ago and often ribs me about continuing to work.

'No-one goes to their grave, Peter, saying they wish they had spent more time in the office!' he quips.

'But Paul, as a colorectal surgeon, I work up an orifice not in an office!' I counter while reminding him that I still also enjoy it a great deal.

One of the surgeons who works for me is now seventy-three years old. He has a little tremor but operates very competently and safely. I keep a gentle eye on him. He was forced to retire at sixty-five before the rules changed.

'I just got so bored, Peter!' he told me. 'Luckily I was able to come back to do about three days a week. I love it.'

Therein lies an important message. It applied to me. I was able to reduce my more difficult commitments by pulling out of management tasks and giving up the heavy lifting of treating the colorectal cancers and dreadful major abdominal catastrophes. By taking this decision, I was able to side step the stresses of administration on the one hand, and those serious clinical complications on the other. Today most of my work is daycare surgery, so the stress is low and the worry of looking after ward inpatients does not impinge on my life at all. Not quite so thrilling, but more comfortable for an old codger like me.

Of course, government treasurers want us to work for ever and die a day after retirement so they can pay as little of our accrued benefits back to us as possible. I would not want them to have it all their own way but I cannot help admiring those that go on and on. Tycoons still buying and selling companies in their eighties. The BBC's David Attenborough still writing and broadcasting in his nineties. Politicians still speaking in the hopelessly overcrowded House of Lords as they near one hundred. Old vicars giving sermons. Musicians touring the world in rock bands with their carers. Even the Queen still working hard at ninety-four.

Work for them is still fun.

Like a good game of chess.

Why would they ever want to stop?

When I Googled the oldest surgeon in the world, I found Alla Illyinichna Levushkina, who is 89 years old. A surgeon at the Ryazan

City Hospital near Moscow. She still performs four operations every day. The article extols exuberantly:

This incredible old woman has been a surgeon for a whopping sixty-seven years, and, although she's already performed more than 10,000 operations, she has no intention of slowing down.

'Being a doctor isn't just a profession but a lifestyle,' she told a reporter.

One of my old bosses is still researching and attending conferences in his eighties and his wisdom is still being appreciated all over Europe and the world.

An extraordinary achievement.

An exceptional life.

But I doubt I will have either the stamina, or the good luck, or reputation, to emulate him.

***

A look into the future is hard. Medicine and surgery have changed so radically in the two hundred years since Lisfranc removed his patients' rectal cancers in conditions we now consider barbaric. Today it is a smooth, humane, routine activity in countries that can afford the manpower, infrastructure and the equipment needed. But there is still much to do to level out the provision of surgical care. Inequality of surgical services around the globe is marked.

But, apart from the poor access and the waiting time in Britain's NHS, I beg forgiveness when I paraphrase the late Prime Minister Harold MacMillan, when I say: 'We patients have never had it so good.'

***

Things change steadily in health care and social understanding.

Humans have such short memories.

What we know today was not so just yesterday.

When I was a young doctor I had never heard of HIV, paedophilia, eating disorders, transgender, child abuse, self-harming, mad-cow disease, Ebola, SARS or Covid-19 pandemics. These are newly described entities. How many other new concepts will we see in the years to come?

In the early twentieth century, Western society dabbled with eugenics but was frightened by what it implied and so retreated. But soon we may have to look again. Debates on when life needs to be allowed to end should be more sophisticated. Euthanasia, or passive medicine, in all its forms must be part of political debate. Until now British politicians have shied away from exploring these subjects leaving them to others to be the pioneers, such as in Switzerland, Oregon and Holland.

Even the recent debate about how we measure the cost/benefit of Covid-19 interventions failed to conclude that life-years-saved was a more important measure than lives-saved. In other words, sparing the life of a five-year old rather than a grand-mother of eighty-five years is a much more significant gain than the converse. That much is self-evident but many do not see it that way.

With regard to my profession there will be even more rapid progress in the years to come. The Royal College of Surgeons of England put out a couple of years ago a useful report about the future of surgery. They concluded that robot-assisted surgery, data analytics, artificial intelligence, genomics, regenerative medicine, virtual and augmented reality, and 3D printing and planning would push surgical frontiers forward.

Whatever the future brings it is clear that young men and women, let us still call them surgeons, will be needed to work those robots, analyse that data, control the artificial intelligence, steer the genomics, target the regenerative medicine, understand the augmented reality and marshal the 3D printers.

But that is the future.

I have only memories of the past and a modest understanding of the present.

I have had my share of fun as a surgeon.

Indeed, I count myself lucky that it has been my privilege to treat patients with problems that I could ameliorate with surgery as it was, and is now.

I have been delighted to see on my patients the smiles on their faces when they went home cured or palliated.

Mostly from the monstrous concrete edifice that is Northwick Park Hospital in Harrow.

That has always been this doctor's aim.

Epilogue

I wrote this memoir during the lockdowns of the summer of 2020 and the first months of 2021. For much of that period during the first and second waves of Covid-19, I worked half-time. Routine surgery ceased for a while, so I found time to reflect.

Living in our rural paradise that is our slice of Hertfordshire was not a hardship. We were lucky.

The family were confined alongside us and, despite the misery for many in the world, it was a very happy time.

We cooked and played tennis. We went for self-distanced bike rides and walked our dogs Rio and Hooch and when Rio died suddenly, we found another puppy who we called Mack.

My work in the hospital was intermittent. Telephone clinics here, operating lists there and virtual teaching sessions on and off.

My horse Galway was a particular joy. Nothing gave me greater pleasure than riding beside my wife Christina, on her Welsh cob, or riding alone on a perfect summer evening. Strangely there were many such beautiful evenings that summer.

On one such evening in late July, I headed out, west along the bridleways. Alone, riding down towards the Valley of the River Chess. It was a fabulous evening. The light was flickering through the hedgerows of hawthorn and the handsome beeches on the chalk hills were spreading their vast canopies over the earth beneath them.

Galway and I found ourselves on one of our favourite bridleways beside a high-hedged, deep-set country lane. We started to trot and Galway picked up his usual sharp pace.

Rising and falling in the saddle as the sun began its descent.

Alone with a horse in rural England.

Unadulterated pleasure.

Suddenly Galway spun round. Like all horses deep in his stone-age psyche, he believes that at any moment a sabre-toothed tiger will attack him.

Instead it was a pair of cyclists in black lycra whizzing in the twilight through the lanes towards him. Like a pair of rapiers ready to run him through.

As Galway spun, I was high in the rising part of the trot. One moment I was on a horse. The next he was not under me. He was twenty feet behind. I hit the turf. My right shoulder took most of the force of the fall.

I was winded. Not hurt. Only my pride was bruised.

I began to walk back to the farm where Galway had run for protection.

At that moment I had a vision of being in a hospital bed.

Like Christina had been six years ago, when she had broken her back falling from a horse.

Now I was the patient.

Now other doctors were fussing over me, just as I have spent nearly half a century fussing over others. They were speaking gravely of how I might benefit from this or that intervention.

Perhaps soon, they would switch off my life support?

Finally the doctor, the surgeon has become the patient.

The medical cycle of life has completed its journey as it inevitably does.

I am now where we all will end.

Awaiting help from those that care.

At their mercy.

I trust they have compassion.

I must have faith in their wisdom to make the correct choices on my behalf.

Just as I have tried to make the right decisions for those who entrusted their care to me these last fifty years.

Acknowledgements

As a surgeon who scribbles I am used to sticking my neck out and upsetting colleagues. As the Americans say, it comes with the territory. Wherever possible I have been truthful as I have retold the stories that have been relevant to my life as a surgeon. Names of colleagues have been changed only when they appear in a poor light. Patient confidentiality has been fully respected, as is the law of the land, though many of the brave men, women and children who I have treated would, I am sure, not be worried one bit if the world could know of their individual acts of courage.

My thanks to the following who commented most constructively on first drafts of chapters: David Sellu, Zora Cass, Barry Cockerell, Tahir Hussain, Neville Robinson, Bruce MacFarlane, David Cox, Sarah Weldon, Alex Tapner, Steven Root, Dave Straton, Helena Bridgeman, Nigel Loli, Jonathan Winehouse, Octavia and Christina McDonald, and my thanks to Andrew Kirshen for his most gracious introduction. My thanks to James Chester and Hooked Books for their helpful advice.

Printed in Great Britain
by Amazon